Colleague Reviews for
"Hey Doc": Memoirs of a Rural Physician

"I read this book with great interest and the occasional tear. In telling a life and career story, Dr. Damos gives us many perspectives—personal, family, medical care, educational, and more. He also notes the impact of the changes in the health care system—and financing systems—on rural practice as well as medicine more generally. Modest about his accomplishments, honest in discussing the challenges, but always passionate in his commitment, this book should be read by all who value family stories, medical care, and rural life."

John Beasley, MD
Professor Emeritus
University of Wisconsin
Department of Family Medicine
Co-concept Originator and Developer
Advanced Life Support in Obstetrics (ALSO) Course

"There was a time during my fourth year of medical school that I had severe doubts about pursuing family medicine as a career after spending much of my training in large urban hospitals. I was fortunate enough to meet an individual who encouraged me to "go to Baraboo, Wisconsin, work with Jim Damos, and he will show you what family medicine is meant to be." I took that advice, and it changed my life, leading me to a wonderfully rewarding career as a family physician.

"This book invites you to ride along with 'Diesel Damos' as he takes you on a journey through his career as a physician. Along each stop, there are new challenges, rewards, and revelations associated with practicing family medicine, all while revolving around the importance of connections with family, friends, and patients. The real bonus of practicing family medicine is being invited into another human being's life, earning their trust, and making a difference by listening, caring, and working together toward a common goal. I would encourage every medical student to read this book to remind them what they are working toward. Dr. Damos, through the many stories shared, truly captures what it means to make a difference both inside and outside the family physician's office."

Jamie Kling, DO, FAAFP
Clinical Assistant Professor
UW Health
Portage, Wisconsin

"Hey Doc"

"Hey Doc"

Memoirs of a
Rural Family Physician

James Damos, MD

E. L. Marker
Salt Lake City

Published by E.L. Marker, an imprint of WiDo Publishing

WiDō Publishing
Salt Lake City, Utah
widopublishing.com

Cover design by Steven Novak
Book design by Marny K. Parkin

ISBN 978-1-947966-18-5
Printed in the United States of America

Contents

Academics and Teaching

Teaching and Practicing Rural Medicine

Introduction

DESPITE NATIONAL EFFORTS TO COMBAT THE problem, there continues to be a shortage of physicians in small-town America. Approximately twenty percent of Americans live in rural areas, but only nine percent of physicians practice there. There is a growing maternity care shortage in many smaller communities across America. Family physicians comprise just fifteen percent of the U.S. outpatient physician workforce, but they provide forty-two percent of the care in rural areas.

General surgeons, internists, pediatricians, mental health practitioners, and orthopedists also offer services in these smaller communities, and they are very much needed. Obstetricians rarely locate in smaller towns, and family physicians and nurse midwives do most of the obstetrical deliveries at smaller hospitals.

Who are these rural physicians? They are under-recognized heroes. The challenges they face are vastly different than the challenges faced by their urban counterparts. They can improvise and think outside the box when their backs are to the wall. Most days, they serve their community without the luxury of having daily on-site, readily available specialty backup at their fingertips. They are not in this for fame or glory. These doctors are not the "white coat type" with an army of medical students and residents following them down the University Hospital hallway. They will never be at the microphone in front of the TV cameras, taking credit for performing the latest heroic surgical procedure. They are broadly trained, and they do their best to provide day-to-day care without limiting their focus to one organ or disease. They form wonderful relationships with families over time. These patients are their neighbors and friends with whom they socialize, celebrate, laugh, and mourn. They are likely a community leader. People refer to them as "Doc."

Unfortunately, many of these rural physician heroes are retiring and not being replaced. Medical schools and larger urban medical centers disseminate many myths about a small-town medical practice that ultimately hurts access in these communities. These ideas steer medical students away from primary care and rural medical practice, robbing them of a potentially rewarding lifestyle.

It is not a secret that the style of medical practice is changing for primary care. All primary care physicians will not experience the small town medical happenings I describe in this book. One's locale of medical practice, corporate influence, along with cooperation and competition between physicians will dictate different practice styles for primary care. Broad training in primary care is still needed.

There is increasing specialization in medicine. Some doctors focus solely on one organ of the body like the lung, heart, brain, skin, eye, or kidneys. Some physicians center only on a specific disease or category of diseases such as multiple sclerosis or infectious diseases. Others practice exclusively in hospitals and do not provide outpatient care. Within the surgical profession, there is a similar narrowing of one's focus like being a transplant surgeon or heart surgeon, and within something as small as the eye, we even have retina doctors, cornea doctors and the like. Most of these specialty doctors practice in urban areas at larger medical centers. It would be difficult to support a full-time, narrowly focused, specialty practice in a smaller town.

No doubt narrowing one's focus has led to many scientific advances that are helping people live longer and experience less morbidity. Approximately eighty percent of children with cancer now survive for five years or more. This is a significant increase since the mid-1970s when the five-year survival rate was around fifty-eight percent.

Surgical procedures have become more refined. An appendectomy or gallbladder operation used to require hospital care for five to seven days or more. Now, patients are discharged the same or the next day. Increasing specialization has changed some physician's lifestyles to be more predictable. Most specialty physicians are compensated better than primary care, making their work more profitable and specialty medicine more attractive.

Despite this increasing specialization and scientific advances, all has not been well. In 2017, the Commonwealth Fund (A private foundation that aims to promote a high-performing healthcare system by conducting independent research on healthcare issues) rated the U.S. healthcare system last among eleven developed countries including Australia, Canada, France, Germany, the Netherlands, New Zealand, Norway, Sweden, Switzerland, and the United Kingdom. The indicators studied were healthcare outcomes, access to care (especially primary care), administrative efficiency, equity in healthcare and care process. For this bottom ranking, we pay the highest prices. The United States was the only country without some form of universal healthcare coverage. Other studies from different investigators have arrived at similar conclusions.

In the United States, a robust, competitive, market-driven, business approach to medicine has been encouraged. Competition between organizations and between insurance companies is the norm as patients pay for waterfalls in the lobby, marble floors, beautiful artwork on the walls, rising CEO and other administrative staff salaries, and TV/radio marketing. The pharmaceutical industry has been under fire for the exorbitant cost of drugs. Patients have been desperate enough to travel to Canada to receive their medications. I saw many patients ration their medication by taking less than the standard dose by skipping doses to save money.

Most would agree, competition in the medical market to date has not worked to contain costs. Congress continues to focus on developing an ideal competitive healthcare market. American satisfaction with our healthcare system has declined. Wait times for doctor appointments have risen. People complain their doctors don't spend enough time with them. Many doctors are frustrated because they are pressed by corporate executives for higher economic production (see patients faster-focus on charges) while also being expected to have high patient satisfaction rates. Millions of Americans cannot afford healthcare in one of the wealthiest countries in the world. Lawsuits for malpractice have increased compared to years ago. We need to ask, who are we creating the healthcare system for? Small-town America has been especially affected.

Within our healthcare system, there is something else that is declining: *relationships.* My narratives of the past in this book will emphasize the need for long-term positive doctor/patient relationships with a primary care physician (family medicine, general internal medicine, general pediatrics). A strong primary care foundation is essential to providing better outcomes and more cost-effective healthcare.

Human connection through friendships, a supportive family unit, church, or other organizations is also crucial to a patient's healing. You will see this theme surface throughout this book. These human contacts are amplified in a small town and are critical when patients face a medical crisis. These augmented connective relationships constitute a significant advantage to smaller community living.

I believe our country's lineup of "All-American caliber" physician specialists and our workforce of incredibly talented non-physician ancillary services working together with a consortium of primary care physician "quarterbacks" leading the team can be affordable in the right system. We all know what happens when a football team loses its starting quarterback. A team of "All Americans" at each position can lose.

We need to learn from other countries. I tried to live this team approach in my thirty-six-year career. I hope you enjoy my story.

Rural Medical Practice

Chapter 1

Graduation

IN MAY 1974, I HAD A FEW WEEKS TO GO BEFORE graduation at St. Louis University School of Medicine. The Dean of the medical school called me to his office at noon. I wondered what this was all about. Did I do something wrong? Was I short on graduation credits?

I arrived at 11:45 a.m. to find seven of my fellow student colleagues waiting outside the office: a group who I knew had done well in school. I felt better but still puzzled.

The Dean pointed us to a table of beverages and snacks. "Dive in," he said. "We will get to the nature of this meeting in a minute."

As we chatted among one another, I noted members of the medical school faculty arriving. Over there was the Chief of Cardiovascular Surgery. Sitting down already was the head of the Internal Medicine department. In walked the chief of Pediatrics. The head of Obstetrics and Gynecology arrived a bit late, in his greens. The meeting couldn't be about recruiting. We students had already been matched with our internship positions for next year.

We sat down for a luncheon, and the Dean finally let the cat out of the bag.

"You are probably all wondering why you are here. Well, I have good news. You are now members of a very prestigious society: The Alpha Omega Alpha Honor Medical Society. You were chosen by the faculty, not only for your academic standing in the class, but also your professionalism, ethics, leadership, and the possibility of future success in medicine. Congratulations from all the faculty."

Wow, what an honor!

"Let's go around the room and please share with us what specialty you have chosen and where you will be training," continued the Dean.

I listened to my colleagues tell of entering specialties like Orthopedic Surgery, Cardiovascular Surgery and Internal Medicine with aspirations of becoming a Cardiologist. Someone else planned to become a Gynecologic cancer surgeon.

It was finally my turn. "Well, I am entering a family medicine program. I plan to become a small-town primary care physician,"

After socializing with the faculty, the luncheon ended with congratulations to everyone, and we all began to leave. My student colleagues and I gather outside to congratulate each other and talk further about our future careers.

John says, "Jim, I have a question for you. Isn't general family practice dying? I am told rural family physicians have routine, dull medical practices. Most are triage officers who refer everything to specialists. To me, that would be dull and monotonous. I have heard general practice is not going to be around a few years from now. I always pegged you going into OB/GYN or an internal medicine subspecialty.

Kathy furthers the critique. "I don't think I would enjoy living in a small town. People there can be quite opinionated, closed-minded, and I hear they don't follow the doctor's instructions very well. Besides, the school districts there are not as good. Good luck to you, Jim, but it is just not for me."

I replied, "Well, my wife, Linda, was valedictorian of her small high school and turned out to be an honor student in biochemistry at the University of Illinois in Urbana. I have thought about going into rural practice for a long time now. I want to be broadly trained, which is why I chose family medicine. I know there are health-care access problems out there—not enough doctors. To me, the people appear down to earth, social, and friendly. They seem to value relationships with each other and help each other out in times of need."

John follows up. "I don't know how you can remember everything in each area of medicine. I prefer to focus on one smaller area. Besides, the pay is much better when you specialize. But I too wish you good luck, Jim."

Joe says, "Will you deliver babies out there? My professors tell me lots of women and babies die in small towns because few obstetricians practice there."

Smiling at everyone, I respond, "I am going to do my best, folks. I wish you all well in your future careers. Congratulations to everyone." We shook hands, hugged, and went our separate ways.

That night I drove home wondering if I made the right decision or not. *Oh well, I think I did. Too late now anyway. I am going for it.*

Chapter 2

Our Journey Begins

I T WAS 1977. I HAD COMPLETED MY THREE-YEAR family medicine residency program and was prepared to begin my career practicing primary care in a small farming community. My wife, Linda, and I were in a rented truck on the Illinois Tollway; a peaceful but hot, muggy night with no air conditioning available. Sweat dripped off my forehead. My eyes felt heavy trying to stay awake driving. The radio blared rock music. In the back of the truck, we had furniture and other belongings for three couples, and a blue Volkswagen in tow.

We had graduated from our family medicine residency, two of my fellow residents and I, headed to Reedsburg, Wisconsin, population around 5,000, one hour north of Madison. Reedsburg had just completed a community drive to build a new sixty-bed hospital and clinic and, as a result, was desperate to enlarge their medical staff. They guaranteed us a net self-employment income of $40,000 for the first year.

Linda and I had no money for a down payment on a home, but a bank in town allowed us to purchase a new home with a no money down, adjustable interest rate mortgage as part of the deal. Having spent our adult lives in rigorous medical education, we were not savvy business people. Little did we know what would happen to interest rates. In May of 1977, the prime interest rate was 6.75%. Three years later, it soared to twenty percent, which escalated our loan payments and pretty much tied us into not moving for a while. Perhaps this was clever on the part of this community bank after the town had invested millions in their new hospital.

As I drove, I begin to recap my upbringing in Waukegan, Illinois (population 50,000 in the 1950s and 1960s), in an 800-square-foot apartment with my parents and two brothers. Living in the apartment to our right was my grandmother and aunt. Living in the studio to our left was my uncle, his wife, and two children. To their left was my other uncle, his wife, and daughter.

The family restaurant was downstairs, where they sold hamburgers, French fries, chili, soup, sandwiches, milkshakes, ice cream, and other short-order food. We were a Greek family. The movie, *My Big Fat Greek Wedding,* reminded me of our family. I worked in the family restaurant called the W' Shop, named after Waukegan and the high school across the street. The *Saturday Night Live Greek Restaurant* skit with John Belushi, Dan Aykroyd, and Bill Murray reminded me of my past, as these actors yell out, "cheeseburger, cheeseburger, cheeseburger."

Across the street, many of the high school students would race to eat lunch in our family restaurant when the bell rang to signal the end of the period.

≥▲

I met my wife, Linda Larson, during the second semester of my freshman year at the University of Illinois in Urbana. She walked up the center aisle of the chemistry lecture hall with a load of books in her arms. She wore a flashy plaid dress, sandals, and a bright blue blouse. A plaid scarf secured her long brown hair in a ponytail, which emphasized her beaming smile as she took the seat in front of me. She said hello, and we introduced ourselves. It was hard for me to stay focused on the professor for the rest of the hour.

After several arduous chemistry lectures, I walked with her to the next class we shared, Spanish. With a warm glow, I carried some of those books for her. It impressed me that she shined in both Spanish and chemistry, while also playing clarinet in the Illini band.

I asked her out on our first date the spring of our freshman year where l learned (in a one-hour lesson) how to ride a dorm mate's Honda motorcycle. I had to make a long journey across campus to pick her up at Allen Hall several miles away. I felt so excited and connected to life as I rode across university grounds to greet her. We had fun that evening, and we dated the rest of the year.

We courted during our sophomore year off and on before a disturbing event complicated our future. The pharmacy school at the University of Illinois in Chicago accepted Linda. We were confronted with the typical decision of ranking our continued relationship versus each of our careers: me in pre-med in Urbana and Linda in pharmacy in Chicago. After carefully considering everything through many conversations, I lamented as Linda journeyed to Chicago for her junior year.

Linda excelled in pharmacy school, but the Chicago fires burning all around her in 1968 following the assassination of Martin Luther King Jr. caused her to rethink a pharmacy career.

We were still in contact by phone. The inferno plus our many conversations resulted in Linda returning to the Urbana campus as a biochemistry major. We were married upon graduation from college in 1970. We both graduated with honors, having studied many hours together.

Medical school came next for me, while Linda acquired a job working in biochemistry research at the medical school, and later working in chemistry at the University Hospital in St. Louis.

Linda grew up in Pecatonica, Illinois, a small farming community. The farm she grew up on had been in the family for many years, and everyone, including her parents, sister, and three brothers, worked on the farm. The neighborly town folk would help each other in this rural Illinois community. Linda's father could get to know you in five minutes, and you left feeling he was your long-lost friend. Her mother, a great cook, was a kind and gentle person. When Linda's parents died, at each of their funerals, the receiving line at the visitations went on for up to four hours.

Both of our families were rich in relationships, but neither was wealthy enough to pay for our college educations, let alone medical school. I worked overtime cleaning carpets for a ServiceMaster franchise during the summers and school breaks. I worked during the school year as an undergraduate. Linda had scholarships. We funded medical school through loans and with Linda working full-time as a chemist.

As Linda and I started our new life, the guarantee in annual salary from the Reedsburg community of $40,000 in 1977 was more money than we could imagine, considering our upbringing and having lived on intern/resident wages for the past three years.

After four years of college, four years of medical school, and three years of residency training, finally, at the age of twenty-nine, we were ready to start life. Significantly in debt but hopeful that we could work out of it.

A fellow resident in training with me owned the Volkswagen in tow. Dr. Mike and his wife Lucy had recently had a baby and elected to stay in Lansing, Michigan for Lucy to recuperate and allow the two of them to bond with their new baby. We packed many of their belongings in the truck and their Volkswagen. They planned to join us later driving over in another vehicle. Another fellow graduate from our physician training program, Dr. Bob drove to Reedsburg, driving our car behind us with our beagle dog, Pepper, in the passenger seat. His wife, Barbara, stayed in Lansing getting their affairs in order and caring for their two children. We were all friends and extremely excited to be building this medical practice from the ground up.

We communicated via walkie-talkies as we traveled with our load on the Illinois Tollway.

Dr. Bob called, "Jim, let's take a break. I need gas."

"Okay, let's pull off at the next oasis. We can get out, stretch our legs, take a bathroom break, and try to regroup."

We pulled into an Oasis for gas. I heard Pepper bark as Dr. Bob honked and veered to the right, following the sign for cars. Linda and I, following the sign for trucks, pulled up to the first unoccupied gas tank.

As the dial on the gas tank passed by several gallons, someone came running out of the station yelling, "Hey, you're putting diesel fuel in that truck! They don't take diesel fuel!"

My heart sank. I can't remove all that diesel gas even though in residency I learned how to do blood-letting phlebotomies to treat Polycythemia Vera. I asked the gas attendant, "What now? What will happen?"

"You'll have a rough ride from here to Reedsburg," he said.

I finished filling the tank with regular gas, and we took off from the Oasis. The attendant was right. I couldn't get past thirty mph even with the accelerator floored. The truck acted like a bucking bronco.

I hugged the right lane, with my flashing lights on the rest of the way. Perhaps some calmer music now on the radio? It took us three times longer than anticipated to finish our journey.

As we approached Reedsburg, Linda was motion sick, and Dr. Bob was bored out of his mind from driving so slowly. Fortunately, by the time we reached our destination, the truck began to run regularly again. The diesel fuel had worked its way through, and the engine was now running on the regular gas I added. Dr. Mike and Lucy's Volkswagen had turned from a beautiful blue to black from the soot of my truck's exhaust pipe. It would be quite a job to get that car clean again. This escapade earned me the nickname "Diesel Damos."

Reedsburg, Wisconsin, a small community with friendly people, had an excellent hospital administrative staff. They welcomed us with open arms. The newly constructed hospital was beautiful; the clinic, still under construction, allowed us to help with its design.

Before arrival, we had placed ads for clinic jobs in the local newspaper, seeking prospective office employees. We spent the first-month hiring nurses and other staff as well as purchasing equipment for the office, securing a loan to pay for everything.

The clinic opened for patients the second month. Dr. Bob, Dr. Mike, and I spent the first week sitting at the back of the clinic, playing cards, and waiting for our first patients.

When our nurse came in to announce a patient—"We have a patient here, gentlemen. Looks like he may have a possible strep throat. Who wants him?"—one of us would volunteer to see the patient while the other two held the card hand until the absentee physician returned.

Our card games didn't last long. The local newspaper published stories on each of us, and by the following week, we found ourselves very busy.

Below is a copy of some of our first physician charges in 1977.

Family Practice Associates Fee Schedule

SERVICE	DOLLAR AMOUNT
Brief exam	$8.00
Limited exam	12.00
Extended exam	18.00
Comprehensive exam	35.00
Ear irrigation	10.00
INJECTIONS	
Immunizations	5.00
Allergy injection	5.00 (2.50 each additional)
TB test	3.00
OUTPATIENT SERVICES	
Home visit	25.00
Nursing home visit	12.00
Emergency room visit (8 a.m. to 7 p.m.)	18.00
Emergency room visit (7 p.m. to 8 a.m.)	24.00

HOSPITAL SERVICE

Initial hospital care	42.00
Second-day hospital care	18.00
Third-day hospital care	12.00
Consultation	35.00
Total OB care	375.00
Routine newborn care	35.00
Newborn circumcision	30.00

LABORATORY

Urinalysis	5.00
Throat culture	5.00
Pregnancy test	9.00
Blood test for anemia	5.00

Medical insurance companies were just developing in 1977. They had not yet dominated the market. We did not deal with them. We would hand our patients what was called a "superbill" as they left our examination room. They were told to pay cash at the front desk, and they could send their "superbill" to their insurance company for reimbursement. After all, it was the patient who had a relationship with the insurance company, not us back in 1977. Patients knew what they had been charged for the visit. It was an affordable amount paid in cash (e.g., thirty-five dollars for a complete physical, five dollars for that strep throat).

I felt like I was doing what I had been trained to do. I believed in primary care medicine. I hoped to prove to my classmates from medical school that they missed something by not practicing in primary care medicine.

It seems that we train ninety percent of the doctors to cover ten percent of the medical problems that present to a doctor's office. The cases that appear in the medical school-University environment are the more complex, esoteric, specialty type problems. These referral centers see the ten percent of puzzles sent there by primary care. As medical students encounter complex cancer patients, transplants, high-risk obstetrics, and very sick children, they suppose this is a general medical practice. They don't believe they can learn all of this material and remain proficient.

When a medical student gets out into the community and away from the University, he/she sees that the general physician instead typically handles health maintenance and prevention, immunization programs, minor urgent care, ordinary maternity and newborn care, general pediatric care, and treatment of chronic diseases like high blood pressure, diabetes, and heart disease. In the hospital, the general physician treats common problems like pneumonia, skin infections unresponsive to outpatient treatment, dehydration, and the like.

As I started my first regular job at age twenty-nine, I was excited.

Chapter 3

First Office Christmas Party

N EARING CHRISTMAS, WE PLANNED OUR FIRST office Christmas party. The night of the party, I was the one on call for our medical practice. I anticipated a slow night since the temperature registered twenty-five below outside.

My last patient was a two-year-old child with a cough. As I entered the room, he exhibited the "barking cough" of croup. He had what sounded like inspiratory stridor, or a loud, congested sound on breathing in. The child sat on his mother's lap, the parents looking worried.

"Doctor, he has been like this the past few hours, and he's having more trouble breathing," the mother explained. "He is congested and has had a fever to 101 degrees. We gave him Tylenol an hour ago."

I counted his respirations. He was breathing rapidly at around fifty to fifty-five times per minute; average being twenty-four to forty times per minute for a one- to three-year-old. I note intermittent intercostal retractions (when the muscles between the ribs pull inward). This physical sign indicates that someone has great difficulty breathing.

I became increasingly worried. My pulse rate and breathing rose with the seriousness of this little boy's condition. "I think we need to admit him to the hospital. It is pretty cold outside tonight, and I don't want you to go home, have him worsen, and not be able to get your car started." The parents agreed with me.

I called home. "Linda, I'm not going to make it right away to the clinic party. Perhaps you can catch a ride with someone else? I am admitting a child with croup. After I get him stabilized, I'll join you later." Linda assured me that she would make alternative arrangements like she has done all through my medical school and residency training.

In the 1970s, the standard treatment for croup included cool mist. We placed children in "croup tents," and blew cold vapor into this little gazebo. Theoretically, cool mist moistened airway secretions, allowing them to be coughed up easier. In theory, the cold helped with swelling in the airways. Today, there is little evidence that cool mist is effective. Randomized studies of children with moderate to severe croup have shown no advantage with croup outcomes using cool mist tents. Hospital cool mist tents can disperse fungus and mold if not cleaned properly. Finally, these little childhood shelters placed a barrier between the child and the parent. Today's treatment for croup includes steroids such as dexamethasone and nebulized inhaled adrenaline to improve the child's breathing.

I decided to order soft tissue neck x-rays, looking for a condition called epiglottitis. The epiglottis is a flap of cartilage at the base of the tongue. When one swallows, this fold of cartilage covers the trachea (windpipe), so food does not go into the lung. The epiglottis may swell up when there is a bacterial infection called epiglottitis, making it difficult to breathe. A "thumb sign" is seen in these soft tissue neck x-rays (like a thumb sticking straight up). I also ordered a chest x-ray, looking for pneumonia and a "steeple sign" which indicates a swollen upper airway. The trachea will look like the steeple of a church narrowing at the top.

Finally, I ordered blood testing. Mom stayed with the child throughout the evaluation, serious and fearful as she clutched her child in her arms. I too felt concerned about how the child looked. I accompanied them in the hospital as they went for the tests. Children with epiglottitis can go into laryngospasm. Laryngospasm is an involuntary muscle contraction or spasm of the vocal cords. Laryngospasm would shut off the child's airway. It usually happens if the vocal cords are irritated by water, mucus, blood, or pus.

I felt high anxiety as the child, throughout this period, seemed to worsen. He had increased difficulty breathing, and his oxygen levels began to drop. As the child deteriorated, it was apparent I needed to transfer him to the University Hospital in Madison, Wisconsin, where he could receive pediatric intensive care. We didn't have the resources to care for children this sick at our hospital. I was concerned about epiglottitis as I awaited his x-rays.

I called the University Hospital to speak with the physician on call for the pediatric intensive care unit. I felt a tiny bit of relief when I learned I was talking with the director of pediatric intensive care. My previous experience with him had been that he was excellent at working with outlying rural hospitals. Sometimes, physicians in larger urban hospitals did not seem to understand that rural areas may have more limited resources compared to the higher-tech centers, where the latest equipment and many specialty physicians are readily available. Some consultants can even be arrogant and rude on the phone, not beneficial to the care of the patient.

This excellent physician discussed the case with me, going over all the fine details of caring for this child.

"Jim, is he in the croup tent? Are you giving him fluids? Is he in need of oxygen? Does he have a fever? Do you suspect epiglottitis, a foreign body lodged in his throat, an abscess on his tonsil or in the retropharynx (back of the throat), pneumonia?"

I answered all of his questions.

With the child worsening, I wrestled with whether I needed to examine his airway under anesthesia to see if he had epiglottitis. If he did, he would require me to place an artificial airway—a tube in his windpipe—before his epiglottis swelled enough to occlude his airway or before he developed laryngospasm. Such an outcome would present a risk to the patient in our rural hospital if I couldn't place the tube quickly.

I went down to radiology to examine the x-rays.

Before helicopter transport, the University Hospital had a city bus rigged as a traveling intensive care unit that would travel to outlying hospitals to pick up transfer patients. Alternatively, we would transfer the patient by ambulance, and usually, a physician would accompany them. This approach was not the best solution, as it would take me out of town, forcing another physician to cover while I was gone. Many of the physicians this evening were at the clinic Christmas party.

Since the University Hospital had said they could be up to get the child within the hour with the traveling intensive care bus, I felt better. The x-rays appeared to show no epiglottitis "thumb-sign," and the chest x-ray looked like a "steeple-sign" seen with a swollen upper airway one sees in croup. There was no pneumonia evident.

My relief lasted only until one of the nurses said, "Dr. Damos, the University of Wisconsin pediatric intensive care unit is on the phone, and they want to talk with you." She handed me the phone.

"Jim, due to the cold weather we have been unable to get the bus started. We have a second bus, and we are trying to get this one started, too. We should be on the road within the next twenty to thirty minutes. How's the child doing?"

"Bill, I don't think I can wait. He needs to have an airway established." My anxiety and concern had reached a peak. This child's oxygen levels continued to decline, and he was losing ground rapidly. His airway needed to be intubated and suctioned so he could breathe easier.

"Do what you need to do, Jim. We will be up as soon as we can."

As I prepared to establish an airway in this child, I asked myself what would happen if there were no hospital or physicians in this area? We were one hour from Madison, Wisconsin. It was cold out. Would the parents have felt comfortable with this child barking an increasingly congested cough while in the car on the way down to Madison? Did they have reliable transportation for such freezing weather? What if he went into laryngospasm on the way down?

I phoned the nurse anesthetist on call and asked him to come into the hospital to assist me. When he arrived, we took the child to the operating room, where we sedated him after starting an IV in his arm. I inserted a laryngoscope into his mouth to see if the epiglottis was swollen at the base of the tongue, even though the x-rays had shown what looks like an ordinary epiglottis. Maybe I missed something on the x-ray. I needed to establish an airway in this child anyway since he had such difficulty breathing.

"Looks like a normal-appearing epiglottis, but there is thick pus coming out of his trachea," I cried out as I performed the procedure. I took a swab of the discharge and intubated the child's trachea. I suctioned as much of the thick secretions as I could, a copious amount.

We transported the child back upstairs into our intensive care unit and placed him on a T-tube (moistened oxygen hooked up to the tube now in his windpipe). He immediately calmed down since he had an airway that allowed him to breathe better.

I took the specimen I collected to the lab to look at it under the microscope, the lab tech assisting me. What I saw on the slide (a gram stain) were numerous "purple grapes" consistent with bacteria called Staphylococcus aureus.

I decided to call the University Hospital back to see how they were doing and to give them an update. "Bill, I intubated him and have him on a T-tube. His epiglottis looks normal, but he had a lot of pus coming out of his trachea. The gram stain looks like staph. He is upstairs in our intensive care unit now, and his oxygenation is much improved after suctioning."

"Sounds like you're doing a good job, Jim. We're still working on getting the buses started. Here are my comments. Let's get some blood cultures, make sure you culture those secretions, and let's start the child on some broad-spectrum antibiotics to cover for Staphylococcus aureus. It sounds like he may have bacterial tracheitis."

I had already done these things, but it was good to hear confirmation from him with his vast experience in these more complicated cases.

Bacterial tracheitis is due to a secondary bacterial infection of the trachea (windpipe) In this case with Staphylococcus aureus, it resulted in the formation of pus that acutely obstructed the upper airway, leading to a life-threatening condition.

After going over the case with my consult, I returned to check on the child. He looked much better after I had secured an airway for him and suctioned him. I ordered a post-intubation chest x-ray for tube placement then returned to x-ray to review the film. Everything seemed fine. It was time to talk to the parents and give them another update.

As I discussed with the parents the details of what I had done, in walked Dr. Bill, director of the pediatric intensive care unit at University Hospital.

"Wow, those buses are fast. You're a speed demon," I said.

"No, Jim, they're still working on the buses. I grabbed a taxi cab. Our pediatric fellow oversees the unit while I am gone. I will ride back with the mobile intensive care unit bus when it arrives."

What dedication! I thought. This more experienced physician knew I was just starting out in medical practice. He knew I might need help with a life-threatening situation.

After he examined the child, looked at the slide in the lab, and reviewed all x-rays, he complimented me on the work I had done. Dr. Bill was also very kind in telling the family that the staff at our rural hospital had done an excellent job stabilizing their child.

"The people at this hospital have worked to save your child's life in a very competent manner," he told them. The parents appeared comforted that a coordinated medical team was working together to help their child.

The bus finally arrived. I noted the thick smoke coming out of the exhaust pipe, indicative of the evening's icy, frigid air. The little boy, now appearing stable, was boarded onto the mobile intensive care unit on his little stretcher for the ride to Madison.

I drove home knowing I missed the office party, but I didn't care. I felt a tremendous sense of accomplishment in this case, very proud of my rural hospital staff and thankful to the University of Wisconsin.

I remembered my fellow medical students warning me that as a rural primary care physician, I would have a routine, boring, medical practice because I would refer everything to specialists in today's specialty-oriented medical environment. Yes, I referred this patient, but it was not routine or boring. It was challenging and lifesaving for this child.

Fast forward over thirty years, and I was two days away from retiring. I was in the hospital elevator in Baraboo, Wisconsin, headed up to the second floor to make hospital rounds. A lady entered the elevator, stared at me, smiled, and then said, "Hello, Dr. Damos. Do you remember me?"

I confess I did not, and I apologized.

She said, "It was over thirty years ago that you spent a cold Christmas-season night with my husband, me, and our two-year-old son. Remember, he had bacterial tracheitis? Dr. Damos, he is getting married this weekend!" Her eyes welled with tears. As the elevator doors opened, she gave me a brief but tight hug before exiting the elevator.

This short chance meeting, for me, was the essence of family medicine.

Chapter 4

Treating Friends, Employees, and Public Figures

SECTION E 8.19 OF THE *AMA CODE OF MEDICAL Ethics* states that "physicians generally should not treat themselves or members of their immediate families," because professional objectivity is compromised in those situations. Exceptions are allowed for "short-term, minor problems" or "in an emergency or isolated setting." (Robyn Latessa 2005 Mar;12(3).

The American College of Physicians (ACP) Ethics Manual goes further and states that "physicians should avoid treating themselves, close friends, or members of their own families." Also, "physicians should be very cautious about assuming the care of closely associated employees."

Clearly, a committee with no rural physicians in attendance wrote this. In a small town, many of your patients are neighbors, friends, and employees who would have to travel perhaps an hour or more to receive primary care in a metropolitan area.

I adhered to the rule of not treating family members unless we were out of town dealing with a minor problem. I may have given advice, but I tried to have my family members seek care from an outside physician.

Over the years, however, I treated many employees, friends, doctors, family members of colleagues, and neighbors in the office. It is unavoidable in a small town. I delivered the babies of many people I knew personally, including a fair number of the nurses from the hospital and clinic who I worked with daily. In my office, I had a record of their history, exam, treatment, and any prescriptions written. I treated them like any other patient. If I handled them outside the office or over the phone for something minor, I always pulled their chart out the next day and documented what I had done, to keep a record.

Several of my most rewarding patients were employees, neighbors, and friends. Take, for example, the local veterinarian who came in one afternoon with a sore shoulder and a black eye.

"You look like you were in a fight," I said.

"I got called to this farm because a horse had a laceration on the leg," he replied. "I told the owner to hold onto the horse while I repaired the wound because he might rear up. Unfortunately, the owner let go of the horse, and he reared up. I remember quickly backpedaling and looking up as the horse came down, striking me in the nose and shoulder."

After examining him and having x-rays done, I saw he had a fractured clavicle (collarbone) and a broken nose.

Upon follow-up in the office, the clavicle and nose both healed. Dr. Mike Beisbier became and remains a great friend to this day. His wife, Sally, introduced Linda to downhill skiing; and our families took several ski vacations together, enjoying the fluffy snow of northern Michigan. I became their family physician, and Mike took care of our pets over the years. We conducted the care we rendered to each other professionally in our offices as with any other patient.

Treating neighbors and friends in rural practice is unavoidable but can be rewarding.

I learned early in my career about the challenges one could face in the so-called "small-town fishbowl," no different than problems one might encounter in an urban area.

A priest from another town traveled to see me one afternoon. I greeted him. "Hello, I'm Dr. Damos. It is nice to meet you. What can I do for you today?"

The priest spoke in a soft, monotone voice and appeared emotionless as he looked at the floor. "Well, I'm embarrassed to say that I have a discharge from my penis. It burns when I urinate."

I was tongue-tied for a few seconds on how to proceed with my questioning, but I had to take a sexual history from him. He saved me the time.

"Doctor, I have been going to this massage parlor, and unfortunately I have sinned. I have had sex with women there."

A gram stain of the fluid from his penis revealed what looked like gonorrhea; the culture later proved decisive. I reported him to public health and treated him with antibiotics after checking him for other STD-related diseases and providing him with safe-sex practices education, which he appeared embarrassed to receive.

I tried to get him into mental health counseling, as I knew he felt conflicted about all this. He denied depression, suicide ideation, and alcohol or substance abuse all while looking at the floor. He was wrestling with his chosen occupation and calling.

"Doctor, I know you're trying to help by pointing me toward professional counseling, but I will seek guidance within my church, he replied.

His problem was a painful circumstance to deal with in any community. I saw him one other time with the same problem and again treated him and reported it to public health. Still, he refused a mental health referral, assuring me he was getting help within his own church society.

I never saw him after that. He left the area, telling his parish he was being transferred.

ॐ

Another problematic situation arose when a young man in his twenties came in one afternoon with chronic low back pain. He had recently moved back to the area after growing up in Reedsburg for the first eighteen years of his life. He had worked in his new job now for about a week.

I watched him jump onto the exam table like a gazelle, not appearing to be in much pain. His speech seemed pressured and rapid. "Hey Doc, how's it going. I hope you can help me," he said with a big smile on his face.

"I hope so, too," I replied. After taking a thorough history and inspecting his back, I ask him to stand. He could fully forward flex, extend, laterally bend, and rotate his lumbar spine area. He could walk on his toes and heels. He did not appear to have any scoliosis (curvature of his spine). His reflexes were reasonable, and he had good muscle strength in his legs. He had no shooting, sciatica-type pain going down his legs; no sacroiliac pain and no evidence of psoriasis. (Psoriatic arthritis can present with low back pain in the sacro-iliac region). He had no rash or penile discharge, signs of a condition called Reiter's syndrome where patients get low back pain in the sacroiliac joints. His abdominal exam revealed no mass and his urinalysis was normal. He had no fever, no trouble controlling his bowel or bladder, and all his other vital signs were normal. His weight had been stable (he was thin), and he said his appetite was excellent. I did not do a rectal exam to rule out prostate cancer with metastasis to the spine in this twenty-five-year-old. Prostate cancer at this age was exceedingly rare.

I suggested we place him on some ibuprofen, have him see a physical therapist, and then see me back in a few weeks. I found no evidence of severe disease or chronic disk disease.

Then he asked, "Hey Doc, could I get a prescription for some stronger pain medicine? My old doctor used to give me Percocet. Since I've had this back pain before, he would usually write out for a hundred of them with a refill."

Of course, I had found nothing in my evaluation to justify narcotics. I proceeded to respectfully question this young man about alcohol, substance abuse, and possible mental illness. I explained that anytime someone asked for strong pain medication, it was standard for us to ask these questions.

"Look, Doc, I'm in pain. I need something stronger than ibuprofen. Are you not going to help me?"

"Of course, I want to help you," I replied, "but I don't want to addict you to a strong narcotic when it is unnecessary. I will prescribe a stronger prescriptive dose of anti-inflammatory ibuprofen. Combining it with physical therapy should help. I suggest some ice and, if you like, I will give you a few days off work. I would like to see you back in two weeks for a follow-up to see how you're doing."

At that point, he storms out of the office. He swears at the nurse on the way out, saying, "You work for a real quack doctor here, lady."

About an hour later, I received a call from a pharmacist. "Dr. Damos, there's a patient here with a prescription for Percocet number 120 with a refill. I know your signature, and I don't think you signed this." I refused to authorize the prescription.

I reported this incident to the local police department and later found out my patient was the son of a politically prominent citizen in the community. Although I had done everything right, it was a sensitive issue being a new physician in town and having to deal with the politics of this case, but I wanted to do things by the book. I trusted it would not prove to be my downfall.

His father called me later to the telephone. "Doctor, I am quite concerned that you do not believe my son is having back pain. What kind of doctor will not give pain medicine when someone is in pain?"

I replied, "I do believe he is having pain. I suggest you talk to your son about the details of his problem. I need permission from him to be able to talk with you further. If you like, I'd be happy to set up an appointment for both of you to come in to talk with me, if he approves."

He abruptly hung up on me, almost shattering my eardrum.

The father stayed angry with me until he learned his son had a problem with drugs. With the father's help over time, this patient agreed to receive therapy for drug addiction and paid his dues. The father thanked me and became a reliable referral source and a great cheerleader for my practice. The patient eventually returned to the office also and thanked me for firmly holding my ground, while remaining empathic, caring, and ultimately helping him get into rehab.

With this father's prominence in the community and my new practice, it was a delicate state of affairs. I learned through this case that ice always melts under warmth, even in small towns.

Chapter 5

One Day's Patients

I HAD JUST COMPLETED MY HOSPITAL ROUNDS one morning, arriving at the office to the aroma of fresh coffee. I grabbed a cup and reviewed my schedule for the day.

The first patient was a four-year-old child I had never seen before, a regular patient of one of my partners. As I entered the room, the child was sitting on his mom's lap. They were affectionate—hugging, laughing, and playing games. She greets me with a big smile saying, "Hello, doctor. I hate to take up your time, but I think my son is constipated. His belly looks distended, and he is not having daily bowel movements."

I said hello, made small talk to break the ice like I always did, and got to work by asking, "So how many days in between bowel movements?"

"Two to three days recently. He has had a few fevers, but we chalked this up to a virus or even his constipation. I hear kids can run a fever when constipated."

"How about any vomiting, diarrhea, or stool leaking in the pants," I asked.

"Nope, not at all, just no daily bowel movements and a distended belly."

I pressed on. "Has there been any weight loss, appetite changes, abdominal pain?"

"None," she replied with a smile. "I guess I just need some guidance as to a good laxative program."

When I examined the abdomen of this cute little bambino, I, unfortunately, felt a large mass, fixated and unmovable, a bad sign.

While trying to maintain an expressionless face, I said, "Well, let's look into this. I agree the belly looks distended. Perhaps we can get an x-ray of the abdomen here in the clinic to see if stool is collected throughout the intestine."

My heart sank as I left the room to arrange for the examination. We proceeded with an x-ray of the abdomen. The x-ray confirmed what I feared. There was a large, solid mass, not collected stool from constipation.

Giving bad news is always hard to do. Some doctors will fumble for words or may not know how to approach the situation. We had practiced this scene at length in my primary care training through role-playing and empathy teaching exercises.

I fired the warning shot.

"I am afraid I have some bad news," I said.

The mom lifted her head and looked at me attentively.

"This is not constipation. Unfortunately, the x-ray shows your child has a mass in his abdomen." I showed her the film.

This previously bubbly, happy mom suddenly looked like she had an urge to flee. She hugged her child tightly. In a quivering voice, she asked, "What do you think it is?" Tears welled up in her eyes. Her happy day had just done a 180.

I sat down next to her to make direct eye contact. In a softer voice, I said, "At this point, I'm not exactly sure. What I would like to do, however, is get going on this right away to get some answers. I want to refer him to a pediatric specialist I know in Madison, Wisconsin. With your permission, I will make some phone calls immediately so we can get to the bottom of this. I will have the nurse come in while I'm making these phone calls. She can help you contact anyone else you'd like to call. She will give you a map with directions to where we will be sending you. Is there anything else you need at this time or any other questions I can answer for you? I know this is quite a shock and it is not the type of news I wanted to give."

I made a referral to Madison, Wisconsin. The child was diagnosed with late-stage four advanced cancer. He died that same year after an attempt at surgery, radiation, and chemotherapy by the pediatric oncologist and his team.

I felt so sorry for those parents. I could not fathom what it must be like for any parent to face childhood cancer. I never wanted to do so myself. Physicians have a hard time shedding the knowledge of these cases. I was no different. I felt empty inside.

❧

I was quite behind on my schedule after finding this childhood abdominal mass and arranging for a referral, but it was necessary.

The second person, I thought, would be one I could catch up with on my patient schedule. It was a child with a simple problem, an earache. Little did I know this minor pain was not the simple in-and-out-of-the-room infection I'd anticipated.

After the previous case, it was hard for me to walk into the next exam room and greet such a simple problem in a happy, jovial manner. *Grit your teeth Jim, compose yourself.* I forced a smile and said, "Hello there. I hear someone here has an earache."

"Yes, Doctor, he has had these before. I know an ear infection when I see one, and he has a doozy. He needs antibiotics. He is hurting," his mother replied.

I grabbed my instrument—an otoscope—to investigate the ear. "Oh my, this is very interesting. I can see why you are having pain," I said. "This child has a family of ticks living in his ear canal. I see several baby ticks running around and a giant mother tick attached to the ear canal sidewall."

"What? Are you sure that is what you see," his mother replied.

"I am sure," I said while thinking how far behind I would be on my schedule and how this day had turned ugly.

I got a syringe and irrigated the ear canal. The baby ticks came floating out in the basin. I then grabbed an instrument called an alligator clamp and removed the mother tick from the ear canal sidewall. I was amazed at how cooperative the child was during the procedure. I guessed he wanted his earache to be gone.

His mother watched the tick removal procedure while gasping intermittently with mouth wide open. I gave them some antibiotic eardrops, and mom left the clinic in a daze.

With me now way behind on my schedule, my nurse adeptly kept the waiting room informed of how I was doing for time. Rarely did anyone become upset.

After seeing my next patient who had a rash and sending them on their way with treatment for poison ivy, the emergency room called about a twelve-year-old male brought in with vomiting and a headache. The emergency physician felt it would be cheaper for the family to come to the office for what sounded like a bout of gastroenteritis or, in layman terms, stomach flu. Since we were only five minutes away from the ER through an indoor tunnel, I authorized the child to come directly to my office for evaluation.

While waiting for the twelve-year-old to arrive, I saw the next patient on my schedule: a forty-five-year-old man there for a complete physical exam. I completed his review and sent him to the lab to get his blood tests drawn. *Whew! Nothing complicated about his exam. Maybe things will improve today.*

The emergency room patient arrived, looking dehydrated from vomiting over the past few days. He complained of a headache. There was no fever or stiff neck to suggest meningitis; besides, I was sure the ER doctor would not have sent him over if meningitis was suspected.

"I have a terrible headache, and I can't keep anything down," he said in a soft voice.

I asked, "When did you last urinate?"

"Six hours ago."

His mother, looking concerned, said, "What is strange, Doctor, is that he complains of some weakness on his right side. Weakness worries me."

This one-sided weakness steered me toward considering a neurological examination. He indeed had a faint, one-sided weakness. I looked into his eyes with my ophthalmoscope. As I peered into his eyes, staring at his retina, I noted definite papilledema (swelling of the eye nerve when one looks with a flashlight at the back of the eye). This finding indicated increased intracranial (inside the head) pressure.

As it turned out, this young man had a brain tumor which, fortunately, was not aggressive. This tumor was an oligodendroglioma. Following complete removal of these types of tumors, the chance of long-term survival is nearly ninety percent. He later had surgery in Madison, Wisconsin and survived with minimal disability. His mother was forever grateful. She became a loyal recruiter and cheerleader for my practice.

I finished out the rest of my day and went home. So much for a dull, unexciting day in rural practice.

As I walked in the door, Linda asked, "How did your day go today?"

"Oh, it went fine," I told her. I did not have the energy to go through what I had experienced with my first patients today. Sometimes, you need to decompress silently.

Chapter 6

Two Patients Same Week

IF WE INTERVIEWED RURAL PRIMARY CARE PHYSI-cians, we might find clues to certain diseases. These physicians have a vast amount of experience with their exposure to many different types of illnesses over the years. Because their time is limited to caring for an underserved population with fewer resources at their fingertips, they don't do formal research, and they are not trained to do so anyway. However, these rural primary care physicians may hold the answers to some disease causes and treatments. They are observant and have a broad medical knowledge base.

One day, a cute little four-year-old boy came to see me with his mom.

"Doctor, he's been sick for a week now," his mom explained. "I'm so tired of this diarrhea, vomiting, and fever. He won't keep anything down, and I think he's getting dehydrated."

Her voice gets louder, and she begins to cry. "I am at wit's end. I have been giving him different types of fluids: Gatorade, 7Up, water, and he keeps throwing them up. His diarrhea is terrible and not responding to diet.

I gave him applesauce, toast, yogurt, and rice. He no longer urinates, and he is wearing down. I am wearing down. My boss is pressuring me to get back to work. He doesn't get what life is like for a single mom raising two young children."

On examining this little guy, he looked quite ill. He wore a Green Bay Packers sweatshirt, blue jeans, a cute Chicago Cubs baseball cap, and tennis shoes. Irritable when approached, he whined and turned away from me. Otherwise, he was asleep in Mom's arms. His temperature in the office was 101°, his pulse rapid at 120, and his blood pressure on the low side at 80/50.

I discussed my concerns with Mom. "I agree, he looks sick. Let's admit him to the hospital. I want to give him intravenous fluids and perform a battery of tests."

"Let's do it, Doc," she emphatically agrees.

I wrote admitting orders for her to take over in an envelope to the hospital. I called the hospital to let them know of the admission and asked the nurse to call me with his lab results as soon as they return. I was very interested in his electrolyte panel to see how dehydrated he was, and whether he had an electrolyte imbalance. I decided to give him an initial solution of saline infusion at a bolus dose of 20 milliliters (ml) per kilogram over the first hour (around 360 ml), pending his lab results.

About one hour later, I got his results. He appeared to be anemic (lower number of red blood cells that carry oxygen to the tissues). Surprisingly, his kidney tests were abnormal. His BUN and creatinine tests (kidney tests), as well as his sodium, appeared not to indicate dehydration (pre-renal) but, instead, point to kidney failure.

My heart sank. This mom's life was about to get even more challenging. Her child had symptoms indicating a syndrome called hemolytic-uremic syndrome. I called the University Hospital to have him transferred that same day.

I found out a few days later that he ended up on kidney dialysis at the University Hospital where, unfortunately, he died. The cause of death was hemolytic-uremic syndrome.

Later the same week, another young three and a half-year-old boy came into my office with similar symptoms, almost a mirror case of the one I had just referred to Madison. His labs came back nearly identical, necessitating another referral to the University Hospital. This boy also ended up on dialysis later in his hospitalization at the University. Against all the odds, he lived.

Hemolytic-uremic syndrome is a condition that results in the breakdown of red blood cells (those cells in the blood that carry oxygen to the tissues). The breakdown product of the red blood cell is hemoglobin. These fractured red blood cells clog up the kidneys, leading to kidney failure. It did not seem coincidental that in one week, I had two cases where the cause was unknown. These are rare cases. They both lived close to each other in the community.

Hemolytic-uremic syndrome first appeared in the medical literature around 1955. It wasn't until the early 1980s that an infectious agent was identified. Since then, the cause of hemolytic-uremic syndrome has been found to be due to a strain of E. coli O157: H7 bacteria. One sees these bacteria in such places as contaminated meat or other areas where one is exposed to feces. The symptoms are diarrhea, vomiting, fever, abdominal pain, decreased urination, and looking pale. Because I had two cases within one week and because they were in children who lived in the same general area, I suspected the cause of this syndrome was an infectious agent.

I remember discussing my concern about an infectious agent with the physicians at the University Hospital. They told me the cause of this condition was currently unknown. I'm not sure how seriously they considered my observations. At that time, we "local medical doctors" (LMD's) from small towns were not taken that seriously.

These cases made me realize what I loved about primary care. It was like being a medical detective, gathering clues and diagnosing a patient's puzzle as it first presents. This takes a different skill set than that of a specialist, who uses his/her expertise to treat a complex disease after the diagnosis has already been suspected or confirmed. I did not feel like I was becoming stale and outdated in this line of work like my fellow medical students had warned. The broad medical knowledge base required of a primary care physician was an asset to the patient and me here on the "front-lines."

Chapter 7

End-of-Life Care

IN A PEER-REVIEWED JOURNAL, *AMERICAN FAMILY Physician,* February 15, 2017, volume 95, number 4, page 215, under policy and health issues in the news, there is a paragraph outlining a study from the Graham Center. This study states that more primary care involvement improves end-of-life care. The paragraph states:

> Researchers at the Robert Graham Center found that patients in regions with more primary care involvement experience less intensive end-of-life care. To determine the level of primary care involvement, researchers calculated the ratio of primary care physician visits to subspecialist visits. In regions with a high proportion of primary care visits, patients at the end-of-life recorded fewer intensive care unit (ICU) visits, less fragmentation of care, and lower overall Medicare spending. (Claire K. Ankuda 2017 Jan; 15(1))

I agree with the findings of this study. I can illustrate this in several cases.

A patient I will call Joe, in his eighties, came into our rural emergency room one afternoon. He had difficulty breathing. The emergency room doctor made a diagnosis of acute pulmonary edema (fluid in the lungs from a failing heart).

The doctor called my office. "Jim, you better come over. Your patient does not look good. He may die. The family is here."

Minutes later, I arrived at the ER. My nurse, as customary, let our clinic patients know I had been called out for an emergency. She gave them the option of waiting or rescheduling if one of the other doctors or nurse practitioners couldn't see them in my absence.

Joe and I knew each other well. I had seen him in my office over the years for hypertension and high cholesterol. Recently, I had encouraged him successfully to quit smoking.

Over the past few years, Joe had suffered two heart attacks. His heart muscle was already damaged; he now was on oxygen. Before I arrived, the emergency room doctor had given Joe an intravenous diuretic called Lasix (trying to make him pee out that fluid from the lungs) and had given him morphine, aspirin, and nitroglycerine. I noted a urinary catheter hanging from his bed with urine trickling into it.

Unable to speak due to air hunger, Joe gave a glimmer of a smile from his serious-looking, perspiration-soaked face as I walked in. He grabbed my arm tightly with his right hand. I smiled at him and placed my hand on his, reassuring him. In this time of crisis, Joe saw someone familiar who knew him personally. Because of my track record with him, he trusted me. We had a bond.

Joe's smile was not the same one I had seen at social functions or around town through the years. Unfortunately, I had discovered a week previously that Joe also had metastatic lung cancer. A nodule had shown up on a chest x-ray, and he had a lung biopsy positive for cancer. His liver tests were abnormal.

After talking with and examining Joe in the emergency room and after reviewing the studies the ER doctor had done, I wandered out to the emergency waiting room to speak with his family about advanced directives. Joe was dying. Joe's cancer diagnosis had come suddenly. I had not yet had time to cover advanced directives with him in the office. Did he want to be resuscitated? Would he want to be on a respirator? What goals or unfulfilled life events might he have in mind? Joe, in his eighties and very sick, could not talk with me about this now with his air hunger. I needed to discuss these issues with his family.

Joe's wife, who I had followed for diabetes and high blood pressure, sat before me in the waiting room. Next to her sat their daughter, who I had seen for women's health issues over the past several years. I had delivered one of her babies. On the floor, in the corner, sat three of Joe's grandchildren, who I had seen for well-child care, sports physicals, and immunizations. I had sutured a laceration in one and cared for a sprained ankle in another.

It took me ten to fifteen minutes to discuss Joe's condition, explaining the risks, benefits, and alternatives. After hearing their opinions, I recommended how far I felt we should proceed with Joe's treatment. Why only fifteen minutes? Because I had a trusted primary care track record with the family.

I have seen, in my thirty-six years of medical practice, the importance of having a positive doctor/family relationship and having patient continuity of care. If the same case occurred in a hospital where Joe and his family did not know anyone and where the doctors were more distant, the family would experience more distress than they did here.

The care might be competent, but the family feels alone. I saw it throughout my career. These families, when confronted with decision-making by strangers, tend to ask what I call the "suspicious questions" in cases like Joe's.

What kind of doctor are you again? I am not sure I understand you.

Could we get another opinion from another physician first?

I better call Uncle Harry in Indiana to discuss your proposed approach. Can I make a call? I don't know what to do.

Are you sure you have the right diagnosis?

As an expression of their anxiety, some families will express anger toward the medical staff and criticize the medical care. Later, they may seek legal consultation about a malpractice suit even though they had received competent medical care. A frivolous lawsuit may occur because they felt the need for a scapegoat.

What the family is telling these doctors is that they don't entirely trust them. They don't know who these doctors are, nor are they familiar with the other three doctors who have been in to talk with them in the past two hours. These different physicians may have said things to the family perceived as conflicting. I have seen some doctors send their nurse practitioner or physician assistant in to talk with the family instead of going themselves.

In urban, more specialized hospitals, the patient's primary care physician is often not involved in hospital care. In cases like this, when hospitalist physicians (physicians who specialize in hospital care) are caring for a dying patient, it should be mandatory to consult the person's primary care physician. Reasonable compensation for this consult by the primary care physician should be standard. This consultation, in my view, would be welcomed by the family.

Another end-of-life care case depicted the advantages of having a "quarterback" primary care physician (in this case family medicine or internal medicine) who had a long-term relationship with the patient and family.

Harry came in to see me with a swollen right leg. On exam, his right leg looked about twice the size of his left leg. Dilated veins showed through the skin. Further testing revealed a blood clot in his leg. I admitted him to the hospital to get him started on blood thinners, standard care back then. In today's world, conventional care might be outpatient care of this problem, which is much cheaper.

I interrogated him. "Harry, have you injured your leg at all? Have you recently taken a plane trip or a long car ride? Is there any family history of blood clotting?"

"Well, Doc, I recently lost my appetite. I lost maybe ten pounds without trying. I have had stomach upset and pain right here (upper central abdomen) going through like a knife to my back."

Blood testing revealed elevated liver enzymes, and further imaging studies of his abdomen, unfortunately, showed a pancreatic mass. By further studies, this proved to be a pancreatic adenocarcinoma.

According to the American Cancer Society in the 1980s, the one- year and five-year survival rates with all stages of pancreatic adenocarcinoma was poor even with treatment. Poor survival relates to the fact that in only twenty percent of the cases is the tumor confined to the pancreas at the time of diagnosis, allowing a possible curative surgical treatment called a Whipple procedure. Pancreatic adenocarcinoma is hard to discover early in the game.

I sat down to talk with Harry further. I use the pneumonic "SPIKES" in these situations where a grave diagnosis will be shared with the patient.

This pneumonic—how to inform patients of a severe diagnosis—is found in the palliative care literature:

Setting, Perception, Invite, Knowledge, Empathy, Summarize.

SETTING: The setting should be private, with no phone calls. I turned off the beeper.

PERCEPTION: I said, "Harry, what is your perception of what is going on?"

Harry replied, "I know I have a blood clot in my leg, and I'm on blood thinners. I had a scan of my abdomen, and that showed a mass in my pancreas."

INVITE (how much do they want to know): "Harry, you are correct," I said. "So, people are different. Some prefer to know all the details about the diagnosis and treatment of their case and others prefer I talk with a trusted relative or friend about their condition. Which type of person are you?"

It was only in my extremely older patients or ones who were mentally challenged that I was told to talk to someone else about the diagnosis, treatment, and prognosis. Harry wanted to know everything.

KNOWLEDGE (sharing my understanding of the details): I continued, "Harry, I have some bad news. (Fire the warning shot). Unfortunately, this pancreatic mass we found has proven to be pancreatic cancer by all our tests. This cancer has already spread to the liver. You developed a blood clot because people are prone to blood clots when they have cancer. Harry, the prognosis for pancreatic cancer is not good. However, even though the statistics are unfavorable, miracles can occur. I can refer you to an oncologist who is a cancer specialist who will go over different options with you."

"You know, Doc, I had a friend with pancreatic cancer, and he did not do well," Harry said. "He lived only a few months. I know the cards are stacked against me. I have read about this cancer before. I'm not sure I want to see the oncologist. He'll recommend I take chemotherapy. I saw my friend try this and he got very sick. I'm not sure I want to live the last few months of my life throwing up and having other symptoms, especially if it's unlikely chemotherapy will cure me."

EMPATHY: "Harry, I am so sorry to have to give you this news," I said. "Are you sure you don't want to at least to talk with the cancer specialist about your options?"

"Nope, I don't want the referral. If I change my mind, I will let you know."

I couldn't argue with him. In my experience, the oncologists I worked with often suggested a chemotherapy trial to see if there was a response. Rarely, did they discuss prognosis unless the patient aggressively pressed them for an answer. They would share chemotherapy side effects with the patient, but almost always seemed to encourage a trial of chemotherapy.

Harry rightfully felt this would be the suggestion to him based on his friend's experience.

Oncologists use chemotherapy in cases of advanced cancer for two reasons. One, to cure disease; the second, to prolong life but not cure. Oncologists use the term "palliative chemotherapy" to mean life prolongation but not cure. In my experience during the 1980s, chemotherapy for pancreatic cancer always appeared palliative, not curative.

SUMMARIZE: I continued, "Harry, if you change your mind about seeing an oncologist, please let me know. In the meantime, I would like to cover a few other things with you to summarize. You have a blood clot in your leg being treated with blood thinners. You have pancreatic cancer spread to the liver. Unfortunately, this does not have a good prognosis, but miracles happen. You have elected not to see the oncologist. A few other things to think about—first, do you have your affairs in order? Do you have a will made out?"

"Yep, I do. That has all been taken care of."

"Good for you, Harry. I am impressed. Have you heard of the Hospice organization?"

"Yes, I have, Doc. My friend was in Hospice. It's a wonderful organization, and I would be interested in it."

"Good, we will make a referral. I will give you some patient education material on Hospice before you leave. Harry, with the cards stacked against you, do you have any unfulfilled life events you would like to get accomplished? A so-called bucket list?"

"Doc, I have a few," Harry said. "My brother and I haven't spoken to each other for years. I want to patch things up. I am an avid bass fisherman. I'd like to take one final fishing trip. I can't do that if I'm sick on chemotherapy. Finally, I want to spend time with my wife and take a nice long vacation with her. We haven't done that in years."

"Well, let's plan on it."

I continued, "Harry, I also want to tell you I will be in there pitching with you all the way. We've been together too long for me to do otherwise. I will plan on aggressively managing any pain you have; and we will treat such symptoms as nausea, fatigue, reduction in appetite, or any other symptoms you may have. I am very aggressive at trying to maintain comfort with my patients. I work quite well with the Hospice personnel. If you are not planning to fight this tumor aggressively, my recommendation would be for us to establish an advance directive that states you do not want CPR done in case of emergency, but instead, be kept comfortable."

"In the future, any treatment plan we consider should have an end goal in mind. For example, you may wish to undertake full CPR despite your condition if your goal was to attend an important upcoming event; a daughter's wedding, for example. Nothing is etched in stone. You can change your mind anytime. This plan is dynamic and not static. How do you feel about this?"

Harry replied, "I would agree—no CPR at this time."

We stabilized his anticoagulation (blood thinning) program for his blood clot in his leg and controlled his symptoms of pain and mild nausea.

Several weeks later, he visited his brother, they made up, and the two of them went on a final week-long bass fishing trip together. Harry said it was the best trip of his life. After rechecking his blood thinning program, he and his wife then took a one-week vacation together out West. They had wanted to do this for a long time.

They returned home and came into the office to tell me about their successful trips. Harry now wanted to stop all medications.

"Doc, I can't tell you how much we appreciated your honesty in answering all our questions anytime we had concerns. You let us be in control after being honest with us. We understand that the last chapter of our life book is about to close. We have had a wonderful time over the past several weeks. Thank you so much."

They understood I was not acting as a "death panel," as some politicians refer to it, but instead as a human being desiring to see Harry make his own decisions after knowing all the facts.

Harry died one month later. I attended his visitation, and the family again expressed their gratitude to me. They were surprised I had come to pay my respects. They told me they had never heard of a doctor attending a patient's visitation.

Perhaps palliative chemotherapy would have given Harry more time, but this was not his choice. I learned from Harry that truthfully providing patients with all the needed information, allows them to make an informed decision best for them.

After this experience, I became even more convinced that close, long-term doctor/patient relationships are not as overrated as many in the medical establishment claim.

Chapter 8

Diversity of Challenges

ONE EVENING AT SIX, I CONDUCTED AN EXAM in the hospital newborn nursery on a baby I had recently delivered. The labor and delivery had gone well and without complication for this infant. I learned early in my medical career that, most of the time, childbirth resulted in the creation of life, joyful tears, proud parents, and the formation of a new family unit with its exciting potential.

As I examined the new arrival, a nurse approached. "Dr. Damos, would you mind looking at another little guy here? He's not your patient but, to me, this newborn looks quite jaundiced. I know you're on call tonight, and you want to get home to eat, but I'm concerned."

I learned early in my career to trust experienced nurses, who spend much more time with the patients throughout the day than we physicians do. I took her suggestion and examined this baby further.

"You know, I agree he is jaundiced. I will order a bilirubin test," I told the nurse. During my exam, I also heard a heart murmur as I listened to the chest with my stethoscope. *Not good.*

The blood test returned. Normal bilirubin in a newborn might be around 5 mg/dl. This infant's bilirubin returned in the thirties, indicating severe jaundice or yellow skin, which was obvious looking at him.

While still on call, I contacted the family and shared my findings with them, mentioning severe jaundice and the fact that I'd heard a heart murmur. We transferred the infant to Madison, Wisconsin, that evening where he was found to have congenital heart disease. Later, he underwent heart surgery and, after many other operations over several years, the child died.

I felt terrible for this family. Again, I could not fathom how parents could deal with severe illness and death in a child. Critical disease in children was the most challenging part of my job.

Years later, this father wrote me a touching letter. In it, he said that my discovery of his child's congenital heart disease that evening in the nursery provided him and his family with several wonderfully productive years with their son before he died. It was one of those letters that choke you up when you read it. The father didn't have to write this, but something years later must have triggered him to do so, like a birthday or other significant event. I much appreciated this man's gesture, sharing his thoughts with me in such a genuine, meaningful letter.

These cases are hard for any physician to shed. I never seemed to get over occurrences like the adolescent with the brain tumor, the child with late stage 4 cancer who died, the children with the hemolytic-uremic syndrome, and this child with congenital heart disease. I felt so sorry for these parents as their tragedies played out. It hits one harder in a small town since I also knew some of these people outside the office.

꙾

You never know what you will see in primary care. Pneumonia was a typical hospital admitting diagnosis in my small-town practice.

It was mid-afternoon as a fifty-year-old male visited my clinic. "Doc, I've had this cough," he explained, "and my temperature is running around 100 for the past several days. I feel achy all over."

"Well, that's no good. Let's take a close look at you." I examined his eyes, ears, nose, mouth, and throat, and listened to his lungs and heart. I didn't find anything of interest. His temperature in the office was 99.6.

"I think this is likely a viral upper respiratory infection," I told him. "I'll give you a patient education handout on how to approach this conservatively, and it should run its course. Give this a few days, and if you're not getting better, I want you to call me back or make a follow-up appointment."

He returned several days later with worsening of his cough. I ordered a chest x-ray in the clinic, which showed an infiltrate in his right lung consistent with pneumonia. I placed him on oral antibiotics, after giving him an initial dose of an intramuscular antimicrobial to get things going. I sent him home with instructions to follow up in a few days. I felt I could treat this as an outpatient (so-called "walking pneumonia").

He came in for follow-up and reported that he was about the same. I suggested admission to the hospital. He did not seem to be improving, and I thought intra-venous antibiotics might help.

"Doc, maybe I can stay home for a little longer. I would like to see if I can kick this on my own with the use of these antibiotics you gave me. I'm concerned about the cost of hospitalization. I'll call you if I'm no better or get worse."

I instructed him to go to the emergency room that night if he experienced more difficulty breath-ing, became nauseated or dehydrated, or ran a higher temperature.

That night, after dinner with Linda and the kids, I chatted with one of my neighbors as I took out the garbage.

"Hey, Jim," he said, "I was over at my friend's house today. You should see the hobby he has—raising par-rots. His whole garage is filled with parrots."

When he mentioned his friend's name, the light went on in my head. It was my patient with pneumonia! I went inside and called my patient immediately.

"How are you feeling," I asked.

"No different than I did a few hours ago, Doc. I appre-ciate your concern, but you don't need to call me every few hours. I continue to cough, feel achy, and don't feel significantly improved. But let's give it time."

"Well, I just spoke with my neighbor who I under-stand is a friend of yours. He tells me you like to raise parrots. Is that true?"

"Yes, that is true. It is a strange hobby, but it gives me something to do."

"Are any of your parrots sick, by the way?" I asked.

"Yes, three of them have been ill. I've been thinking about calling the vet."

Psittacosis is a disease caused by a chlamydia organism that transmits from infected birds to humans. Parrot disease is another name for *psittacosis*. In humans, the symptoms are fever, chills, headache, muscle aches, and a dry cough. Pneumonia appears on chest x-rays. Endocarditis (heart infection), hepatitis (liver infection), and neurologic complications may occasionally occur. Severe pneumonia requiring intensive-care support may also occur. There are reports of fatal cases.

I again advised admission to the hospital for this bird lover after sharing my concerns with him. There, I treated him with an antibiotic called tetracycline, pending testing (doxycycline had not been FDA approved yet back then). A veterinarian visited his garage and confirmed my suspicions of psittacosis, and my patient's blood test later returned positive for psittacosis exposure. I notified Public Health.

After that case, I added asking about exposure to birds when I took a history of anyone with pneumonia, even though this disease is rare.

Through my exposure to the diversity of challenges that present in small-town primary care practice, I was developing experience in medicine. You never know what you will see in primary care medical practice, and it is fascinating.

Chapter 9

Getting to Know
This Population of Patients

IN CONTRAST TO WHAT ONE MAY HEAR ABOUT small-town America, people are generally friendly, appreciative, and just as diverse as an urban population but on a smaller scale. I would describe the patient clientele from a medical standpoint in three ways:

1. Tolerant, understanding, and often protective of their physician

2. Independent in caring for themselves as much as possible

3. Loyal

First, let's discuss tolerance and understanding. Most small-town patients understand the challenges of a rural physician's daily schedule. For example, if I was called out of the office to deliver a baby in the middle of the afternoon (the hospital maternity ward was a five-minute walk away—three-minute run), most people waited without much fuss. Those who remained greeted me on my return with a smile, often asking me if it was a boy or girl and what the parents had named the baby. Sometimes the waiting room would conduct a naming contest of their own.

Small-town folks are protective of their physician. One summer afternoon in the clinic a farmer named Steve came in for an urgent care appointment, his hand wrapped in a kerosene-soaked rag. I removed the cloth from his hand and noted a swollen, red, painful palm.

"Steve, tell me what happened. This hand looks infected."

"Well Doc, I think I cut it in the barnyard, and it got pretty infected. I would have come in earlier, but I didn't want to bother you right away. You were busy the past few nights. I know for a fact you delivered a few babies this week while you were on call. I listened to the police radio and heard you were heading to the hospital. I put two and two together when I saw the birth announcements in the newspaper. I figured you needed a little rest."

I admitted Steve to the hospital and consulted our general surgeon. He took Steve to the operating room and drained the abscess in his palm. I then placed him on intravenous antibiotics to cover not only gram-positive bacterial organisms (found in a carbuncle) but also gram-negative bacterial organisms (located in a barnyard).

Small-town folks are independent in caring for themselves. One morning I got a call from the emergency room telling me of a needed admission to the hospital. The ER doc said, "I know you are busy in the office, but you need to come and see this."

I finished seeing my last patient of the morning and headed to the hospital. As soon as I walked into the lobby, I smelled a terrible odor.

As I arrived in the emergency room, the scent was unusually pungent. In the ER exam room sat an older man with white hair down to his shoulders and a white beard down to his waist. His fingernails and toenails were long and filthy.

The ER doc warned me that I had not yet seen the origin of the smell. He rolled up this man's pant legs, and I saw jaw-dropping ulcers covering most of his lower legs. Something moving caught my eye; maggots crawled in the sores. These little creatures only eat dead tissue and do not hurt live tissue. Ridding wounds of dead tissue is called debridement. Leg ulcers often are recurrent. This eccentric man did not clean his wounds allowing an army of maggots to gain a foothold. He had learned how maggots helped the healing process and decided to leave them be.

After I did a proper history, physical exam, and ordered labs, the nursing staff took our man to physical therapy to bathe him and cut his nails before admitting him to the medical ward.

The next morning, when I saw him in the hospital, he looked like a new man: clean-shaven, with a haircut, sitting up reading Shakespeare. He was quite intelligent and could quote many Shakespearean verses by memory.

When I arrived at his bedside and began to examine him, he said to me, quoting Shakespeare's *The Merchant of Venice*: "If you prick us, do we not bleed? If you tickle us, do we not laugh? If you poison us, do we not die? And if you wrong us, shall we not revenge?"

The visiting nurses investigated where this patient lived—a one-room cabin with a dirt floor out in the country. His pet dogs ran around inside, unable to get out to relieve themselves. A visiting nurse took them to the Humane Society. He had minimal silverware and almost no dishes or tableware. He cooked his food over a wood stove, threw it on some newspapers on the kitchen table, and ate off that. The next night, he would throw down new papers for his food.

This man spent the winter in the county nursing home, healing his leg ulcers and getting medically "tuned up." When spring came, and the weather improved, he checked out of the nursing home and returned to the cabin. The visiting nurses visited him throughout the summer as much as they could within the constraints of Medicare. They did what they could for him, supporting him in his environment as much as possible.

When the weather turned cold, he again presented to the ER, brought in by the visiting nurses before the winter began. Once more, he was admitted to the hospital, cleaned up, and sent to the nursing home, where he was medically tuned up, and then went home as soon as he looked and felt better in the spring. This behavior became a pattern for him.

I remember another independent man who used goose grease and turpentine on his leg ulcers. This combination is a Southern remedy for colds. Mothers used to mix this at home and rub it on the chests of their children. This man swore this treatment cured his leg ulcers.

Finally, most rural people are quite loyal. When we started our practice, three physicians in town in their upper seventies and early eighties still practiced medicine. They were experienced, dedicated to their patients, and hard-working, although practicing with a style of medicine from years past.

Despite these more outdated practices and the ages of these physicians, they had sizable, loyal patient followings. They had treated a number of these people for many years and had favorable track records with them. Their patients were satisfied. These older physicians resisted retirement, placing us in the uncomfortable position of having to evaluate their standard of practice at peer review. I was on the peer review committee.

As we met on the committee and consulted with the State Medical Society, these physicians began to trust us more. They saw us integrating into the community and not doing harm to anyone. They then, and only then, decided to retire. These older physicians felt protective of their long-term patients just as their patients had shown loyalty to them.

One of these older physicians, and some of the other physician's family members, ultimately became patients of mine. This senior physician had a wealth of fascinating stories.

I used to make house calls on him and, over a cup of coffee, I listened to his stories of the horse-and-buggy days.

One day, he told me a remarkable story. "You know, Jim, I'd like to tell you a story that paints a picture of what us old timers used to do in the old days."

"I'm all ears," I replied.

"Well, one night I got a call to go out to a farm where a woman was having a particularly difficult time with childbirth. When I arrived, I noted she was continually bleeding a slow trickle of blood. I performed a vaginal examination and noted a placenta previa."

A placenta previa is when the afterbirth is low lying and covers the cervix blocking the baby's exit from the womb. He had discovered this placenta previa by doing a vaginal exam. Doing a vaginal exam if placenta previa is suspected is a no-no. A vaginal exam could lead to massive bleeding by dislodging the placenta. In today's world, the doctor will order an abdominal ultrasound in any pregnant woman who is experiencing vaginal bleeding in the last three months of her pregnancy. If a placenta previa is found on the ultrasound, no one should do a vaginal exam. If the pregnancy is mature and the baby is ready for delivery, a cesarean section is performed. Ultrasound was not available back then.

"After I found the placenta previa, I contacted an obstetrician in Chicago, because I knew the patient would need a cesarean section. The obstetrician said he would take the first train up. The patient was losing blood and needed a transfusion. I had her husband get into the upper bunk of their bunk beds with her underneath in the lower bunk. I ran his blood into her with an IV needle and tubing. Fortunately, there was no blood incompatibility, and I think this transfusion saved her life.

"The obstetrician arrived later. We placed the woman on the kitchen table, and I administered ether anesthesia with a handkerchief while the obstetrician performed the cesarean section. We ended up with a healthy mom and baby."

I could not imagine such a scenario. The fascinating thing about this story is that even with these medical practices, which I'm sure had a higher incidence of poor outcomes, there were no lawsuits. *I wonder what the difference is.*

Interacting with these older physicians taught me that I did not wish to practice into my seventies or eighties. I wasn't sure how these physicians did it. What stamina!

And their strong patient followings taught me that when you are kind, dedicated and loyal to your patients, developing a positive relationship with them over many years, they will be compassionate, devoted and committed to you in return.

Chapter 10

Rural Maternity Care

I FELT THAT ATTENDING IN PREGNANCY AND childbirth was one of the most rewarding events in medicine.

A young couple experiences the excitement of becoming pregnant. A stressful nine months follows. Couples experience a full range of emotions and symptoms. Mothers may experience disbelief, self-doubt, fear, and worry throughout the prenatal course. Mothers also experience somatic symptoms such as fatigue, weight gain, abdominal cramping, morning sickness, and other aches and pains. Some fathers develop a condition called Couvade syndrome, where the father inherits some of the same somatic symptoms as a mother (fatigue, nausea, aches, pains, etc.) in almost a sympathy response. Many of these future parents attend prenatal classes which confirms the fact of coming parenthood. The expecting couple will have monthly doctor visits, and there may be imaging such as ultrasound and other lab tests. Such life changes are an adjustment for anyone, let alone a young couple.

The last trimester of pregnancy arrives, with the anticipation of labor and delivery. *What will happen?*

Will our labor be normal, abnormal, painful? The day finally arrives, and the couple heads to the hospital as labor begins. In the end, hopefully, comes the successful birth of a crying baby, parental tears, and a look of relief in everyone's eyes, including the doctor's.

This whole event always seemed a miracle in my eyes. Maternity care became a favorite part of family medicine for me.

Nationally, the number of family physicians providing maternity care has been declining for many reasons. Malpractice, lifestyle issues, lack of role models in residency training, and fear of obstetric emergencies are some of the major causes of this exodus, a trend which hurts access to maternity care in rural America.

Most obstetricians regionalize to urban centers and teaching hospitals. Only about six percent of the nation's OB/GYNs work in rural areas, according to the latest survey numbers from the American College of Obstetricians and Gynecologists. (ACOG).

A study in May 2016 by the University of Minnesota Rural Health Research Center found that in twenty-three percent (almost 1 out of 4) of 244 rural hospitals in nine states surveyed, family physicians were the only clinicians delivering babies at these sites. The regions studied were Colorado, Iowa, Kentucky, New York, North Carolina, Oregon, Vermont, Washington, and Wisconsin.

Low-risk maternity care in rural communities is the primary responsibility of family physicians and nurse midwives, who often practice together. As an example,

I practiced my entire small-town career without a full-time obstetrician on staff at my rural hospital. I did co-practice with maternity care nurse practitioners and nurse midwives.

Should women who live in smaller communities plan on traveling to a larger city and larger hospital to deliver their baby? Nesbit et al. found that local maternity care services may help prevent non-normal birth to rural women and, among privately insured women, might decrease the use of neonatal resources.

One of my first obstetrical deliveries in rural practice was a challenging one. It so happened that I picked up this patient as a new patient in her last month of pregnancy.

Once she became overdue, we had to admit her for induction of labor. Her labor responded nicely to a medication called oxytocin (Pitocin); she progressed to having a fully dilated cervix. During the pushing phase, she complained about a fair amount of back pain.

As I checked her, I felt quite convoluted soft tissue, almost like brain tissue. *Oh, no! Would one of my first deliveries in practice right out of residency training be an anencephalic child that had gone unrecognized?* After having just moved to town and starting my practice, I had only seen this lady for a few weeks in her last month of pregnancy.

Anencephaly is the absence of a significant portion of the skull covering the cerebral hemispheres; it occurs during embryonic development. One will feel brain tissue on the vaginal exam.

I called in one of my colleagues to double-check my findings. He agreed that things did not feel right on the vaginal exam.

On a vaginal exam, it can be hard to determine the position of the baby. We had no ultrasound machine on the delivery floor. I did not feel compelled to order an x-ray when she was beginning to push, and delivery could be imminent.

I was anxious, this being one of my first obstetric deliveries in medical practice. A few minutes later, it became apparent what we were dealing with. As I examined mom again vaginally, I felt an orifice. As I gently explored this hole with my finger, it seemed to suck on my finger. The baby was mentum anterior (chin facing the ceiling) with the face, not the back of the head, presenting in the birth canal. The baby was looking up at the ceiling, the head and neck were extended and not flexed, and it was wrinkled facial tissue, not brain tissue, that we felt.

The exhausted mom had difficulty pushing the baby out. The fetal heart tones became non-reassuring (dropping lower with contractions), so I ended up delivering this baby by forceps. Fortunately, I had been appropriately trained to use outlet forceps when the baby was low in the pelvis and near delivery.

The obstetricians in my residency training program back in the 1970s took pride in making sure "their family medicine residents" knew how to manage delivery room procedures pertinent to rural practice. Obstetricians paged me to the delivery area during my residency training for such things as instrument delivery, manual extraction of the placenta (after birth that was not coming out), and repairs of birth lacerations. I was called to assist on cesarean sections and to help resuscitate babies. This training was essential when considering where I wished to practice medicine.

Baby and mom did well after my instrument delivery, and I developed greater confidence in my new medical practice.

My confidence quickly shattered with another challenging obstetric delivery.

I will never forget the mom from Chicago, a tourist visiting our area who came to our maternity ward while on vacation, in labor with her fifth child. It appeared to me that she had a large infant, but she was progressing with her contractions. Her prenatal records were unavailable. She denied being diabetic. Little did I know that this baby would be one of the most challenging deliveries of my career.

"Come on now, Lila, push with your contractions. The nurse will help you. I can see the head. I think you will deliver in the next few pushes," I said, expecting this to be over soon.

The nurse stood ready to receive the infant.

After a few more pushes, the head slowly delivered over mom's perineum. I note the elongated head and, as it came out, it exhibited what we call the "turtle sign." In other words, the head retracts like a turtle into its shell.

This sign immediately invoked fear and panic in me. I knew this signified the shoulders stuck in the pelvis (shoulder dystocia), and the baby would be a challenge to deliver. It can be a condition that leads to disability and death in the infant.

I began to sweat, working to deliver this baby. "We are going to have a tight squeeze here," I shouted to the nurse, indicating the need for extra help in the room.

I engaged in a series of maneuvers trying to free the tight shoulders, but in the 1970s, this condition had no standard pneumonic or protocol. Textbooks gave suggestions on how to release the shoulders by rotating the shoulders of the baby clockwise and counterclockwise (corkscrew maneuver). It was also taught to have the nurse apply pressure to the top of the uterus (fundal pressure). This is no longer recommended as one can rupture the uterus. Some textbooks taught how to intentionally break the baby's collarbone, causing the shoulders to collapse.

An emergency like that makes minutes seem like an eternity. I had never sweated so much in attempting to deliver a baby. My shirt was soaked. My hands shook, but finally, we freed the baby.

"Let's take the baby to the warmer," I announced as I assessed for breathing, circulation, and responsiveness. The baby laid as loose as a dishrag in my hands, had a slow pulse, appeared blue, and was not breathing well. "Give me that Ambu bag," I added.

We started to stimulate the baby. I suctioned the mouth and began breathing for the baby using the Ambu bag instrument. After maybe thirty seconds, the baby let out a cry and developed some tone in his muscles. Everyone breathed a sigh of relief.

On weighing this infant, the scale revealed a ten-pound baby. Talk about a future linebacker! The nurses swore he growled in the nursery.

I feared what might have happened if our hospital had not delivered babies; and this had happened in the car on the way down to Madison, Wisconsin, one hour away.

One of my mentally toughest obstetric cases occurred one day and into the evening. I had followed a delightful couple for several years. They wanted to start a family, and she, unfortunately, suffered a miscarriage. After a year of trying again, she finally achieved a viable pregnancy, which I followed to the last month.

One morning, I received word that this mom was in our labor and delivery unit at the hospital. She thought she might have ruptured her membranes. She was three weeks before her due date when she noted a limited amount of pink, thin, watery fluid in her underwear.

From the clinic, I ordered an ultrasound exam over the phone, then went over to see her in the maternity ward. There was a healthy amount of amniotic fluid, one baby with the head presenting (not breech), and no placenta previa reported on her ultrasound. These findings were reassuring. I performed a sterile speculum vaginal exam. During my vaginal exam, I saw no pooling of fluid in the vagina to suggest she had ruptured her membranes. Her cervix was closed. Everything appeared normal.

The fetal heart tones on the fetal monitor reassured me, as did a non-stress test of the fetal heart tones. The fetal non-stress analysis showed the baby kicking with good accelerations of the fetal heartbeat during the kicks, a good sign. When the fetal heart goes up fifteen beats/minute for fifteen seconds after a baby kicks, and this occurs twice in twenty minutes, that is a sign of fetal well-being.

I had her walk around with a pad on for several hours, and there was no leakage of fluid noted. She had no contractions. We discussed the possibility of induction of labor, but since she was still three weeks before her due date, I discouraged this. Also, she had an unfavorable cervix for induction of labor. She wanted to do things naturally, and I agreed.

Today it is considered better to induce someone closer to one week before their due date rather than fifteen to twenty-one days before, although pregnancy is regarded as a term pregnancy after thirty-seven weeks in a forty-week pregnancy. If the calculation of the due date is off, it will result in the possible delivery of a premature infant if one delivers the baby longer than one week before the due date.

Later that afternoon, I discharged her, after providing her with patient education on when to return. Perhaps she had some "bloody show." Bloody show is bloody mucus that may pass when the cervix begins to thin (effaces) in anticipation of labor.

I finished in my office and went home for the evening. I was not on call that night. After dinner, I sat down on the couch to read the newspaper.

The phone rang, and Linda called out, "Jim, the hospital needs you immediately."

When I answered, a distressed nurse with a tremor in her voice said, "Dr. Damos, remember the mom from this afternoon? Well, she is undergoing an emergency cesarean section. The baby has been delivered, and they are currently attempting to resuscitate the baby. You are needed right now."

"Gotta go; see you later." I shouted as I ran to my car in the garage. My heart sank as I flew into the hospital.

As I walked into the surgery room, I felt the stress radiating throughout the room. One of my partners was conducting a resuscitation on the baby. The baby had a tube in her trachea, and they were breathing for the baby with an Ambu bag connected to oxygen. CPR was ongoing.

My partner filled me in as I helped him conduct the resuscitation. "Jim, they went home this afternoon. She lay on the couch resting when she felt like she was losing urine. She got up and noted the sofa was soaked with blood. She felt faint when she stood up. Her husband scooped her up and into the car and raced her to the hospital. When she arrived, she was still bleeding, and the baby's heart tones were 30. [Normal being 120.] We went directly to surgery while initiating maternal resuscitation."

Unfortunately, the baby died despite our resuscitative efforts.

I felt terrible. As I walked out to the waiting room to discuss what happened with the family, I tried to compose myself. I felt mentally numb, wanting to retreat inside.

Did I miss something? Am I at fault for what happened? I'm not sure I can stomach that: a life lost because of a mistake I made, especially with these beautiful people who had already experienced a miscarriage and difficulty getting pregnant again.

I approached the fathers' waiting room, where her husband and her parents sat, and I nervously reviewed the whole case with them.

After informing them mom was stable, I fired the warning shot: "I have some bad news. Unfortunately, the baby has died."

The father initially looked at the floor as he sat down overwhelmed. However, rather than breaking down further or becoming angry with me as some patients will, he stood back up and put his hands on both of my shoulders. Looking me in the eyes, he said, "I know you did everything you could."

Composing myself now became even more difficult.

The nursing staff, extraordinarily empathic, gathered the family in the delivery suite with the baby. They were given as much private time as they needed to grieve.

I ordered a pathological examination of the placenta. As I looked at the placenta, it did not appear to have any blood clot to indicate an abruption, or a premature tearing away of the placenta from the uterine wall. However, the umbilical vessels looked strange to me. Again, had I missed something?

I returned home, unable to sleep for days, tossing and turning while second guessing myself. Linda knew

I was hurting. This loss was such a tragedy. I felt terrible for these people.

As physicians, we always second guess ourselves. Some physicians can develop a more hardened attitude to adverse consequences, realizing that perfection in every case will not happen. I had a hard time establishing this approach and was probably overly tough on myself. What affected me even further was the kind and forgiving attitude of this family.

My daily hospital rounds on this case were challenging. There were many concerns about what had happened pending the pathology report. The parents' behavior toward me was always non-threatening and kind. They often followed our discussions by saying: "How are *you* doing?"

A few weeks later, I received a letter in the mail from the parents. Initially, my paranoia made me think they had changed their minds and become angry. This would be the letter informing me of the upcoming lawsuit.

Instead, it was a beautiful letter complimenting the entire obstetrical staff for the care we rendered in these most difficult times. What courageous and kind people.

Later, I received a call from the pathologist, who informed me that the examination of the placenta showed what is called a vasa previa. Vasa previa is a rare obstetrical condition with a reported incidence of around 1 in 2500 pregnancies. In this condition, the baby's blood vessels run near the internal opening of the uterus and are incorporated in the membranes. If the membranes rupture, they may include these blood vessels and the baby begins to bleed.

The diagnosis is often not made before labor. What probably happened was that this mom's membranes developed a small tear into one of these vessels, causing the slight amount of bloody fluid she noted on her underwear earlier in the day. This likely sealed off when she was in the hospital. We documented no blood or leakage during our examinations. The ultrasound exam completed during her admission missed detecting this anomaly, which was difficult to detect in those days.

When she returned home, the tear likely extended, and the blood vessels tore, causing the baby to hemorrhage. When vasa previa goes undetected, it results in fetal death ninety to ninety-five percent of the time. When an ultrasound detects it, a cesarean section is performed, and the infant survival rate is nearly one hundred percent.

This was a terrible case with a poor outcome. I felt no better. My self-incrimination must have shown during mom's follow-up office visits.

One day, Linda and I received a dinner invitation from the parents. With some hesitation, we accepted and went to this couple's home. Upon arrival, we exchanged small talk before the father finally addressed the elephant in the room.

"Doctor, I just want to tell you that we know you and your staff did everything you could to save Catherine, our baby," he began. "We are forgiving people and believe everything happens for a reason. We don't always understand why these things happen, but we don't question God. We know you hurt just as much as we do, and we wanted to reach out further to you. We will never forget you and your staff, and we will always remember Catherine."

Here sat two people who had lost their baby, and they were consoling me? Years later, they came to see me again when they were expecting. I referred them to a high-risk maternity clinic. They had an uneventful pregnancy and a repeat cesarean section with a healthy child, now living in a fantastic home with genuinely beautiful parents.

These people did not fit the myth of rural people being stubborn, opinionated, or problematic.

There were many other maternity cases I encountered during the early practice years that allowed me to develop an enormous amount of experience practicing at a hospital with no obstetrician on staff. I delivered vaginal breech babies who arrived at our hospital in labor before the standard of care changed to cesarean section. I dealt with malpresentations and malpositions of the baby, and preeclampsia or what is called toxemia of pregnancy when referral to high-risk was unavoidable.

Other cases included post-partum hemorrhages, the use of forceps and vacuum instruments, assessing preterm labor, first and third trimester vaginal bleeding, and the delivery of preterm infants who arrived at our hospital with the head crowning from an outlying area. I always tried to refer as much high-risk obstetrics as possible to the high-risk centers and obstetricians in Madison. I knew my obstetrical colleagues had the skills to care for higher risk pregnancies, and I did not try to usurp this talent.

However, many of these higher-risk women in emergency situations would have never made it to Madison. Some of these mothers drove thirty to sixty minutes to get to our hospital (sometimes on snow-covered country roads), let alone having to navigate yet another hour to Madison, Wisconsin while in active labor. For example, if they were being followed in Madison with an obstetrician because of twins and preeclampsia, they might stop at our hospital thinking they may not make it to the city due to intense labor. If our exam noted the delivery of the baby to be imminent, we had no choice but to manage them in our hospital to avoid a car or ambulance delivery of a high-risk pregnancy.

In my career, I delivered close to a thousand babies. Fortunately, I was never even threatened with a lawsuit. Yes, maternity care was indeed a favorite part of my medical practice because I felt my partners and I were desperately needed.

Chapter 11

Emergency

ONE DAY IN THE HOSPITAL, AS I WROTE MY last progress note on a patient with pneumonia, I heard the hospital intercom blurt out, "CODE BLUE, LOBBY OF HOSPITAL. CODE BLUE, LOBBY OF HOSPITAL."

I ran to the lobby, where I saw people surrounding a man on the floor. As I approached him, he looked pale and unconscious.

I shook him and questioned him, "Can you speak? Hello, are you there?" There was no response. He was not breathing, and I couldn't feel a pulse. We started necessary life support procedures, doing CPR, placed him on a stretcher, and rushed him to the emergency room.

While we went through our initial exam survey, I noted that he was a large man with an obese abdomen. He had no pulse or blood pressure, but when we hooked him up to the cardiac monitor, he had a heart rhythm. Having a heart rhythm displayed on a cardiac monitor without a palpable pulse is called pulseless electrical activity (PEA). This condition caused me to go through a differential diagnosis; one taught in the Advanced Cardiac Life Support (ACLS) course.

We proceeded to intubate him to establish an airway, undressed him, got IVs going, and placed a catheter in his bladder. The Advanced Cardiac Life Support (ACLS) course teaches you to think about the 5H's and 5T's in this situation:

H's

Hypovolemia (loss of fluids or blood loss)
Hypoxia (low oxygen)
Hydrogen ion (acidosis)
Hyper/hypokalemia (high/low potassium)
Hypothermia (low body temperature)
     And some say
Hypoglycemia (low blood sugar), although ACLS has removed this from the protocol at the time of this writing

T's

Toxins or Tablets (poison or drugs)
Tamponade (cardiac), or what is referred to as fluid around the heart
Tension pneumothorax (collapsed lung from trauma for example)
Thrombosis (coronary)—a heart attack or
Thrombosis (Pulmonary or lung)—a blood clot in the lung
     And some say
Trauma, although ACLS has removed this too from the protocol at the time of this writing

As I considered these things, I noted his obese abdomen was getting bigger. I wondered if this might be because we had the airway tube in his esophagus instead of in his trachea (windpipe), and we were pumping air into his stomach instead of his lungs.

I listened to his lungs during the artificial breaths; they seemed to be inflating correctly. His oxygen levels had improved. I ordered an x-ray of his chest and abdomen, suspecting he had ruptured an abdominal aortic aneurysm.

Back in those earlier days, we had what was called MAST trousers (medical anti-shock trousers). Introduced into medical practice during the Viet Nam war, they were also named military anti-shock trousers. They looked like a pair of pants. The legs and abdominal segments wrapped around these body parts, fastened by Velcro. After application, they were inflated with a foot pedal to compress the legs and abdomen, thus squeezing blood out of the lower body and shifting it to other parts of the body like the heart, lungs, and brain (almost like an autotransfusion).

Today, their use is controversial, and they are no longer used compared to the 1970s and 1980s. I felt these MAST trousers might put pressure on his aorta and slow down the bleeding. In a rural hospital, we couldn't call a vascular surgeon to come down from upstairs.

I called the general surgeon on call immediately. He arrived quickly, and when he walked into the ER, I reviewed what we had done. He examined the patient, considered the lab results we had ordered, evaluated the x-ray films; and then, surprisingly, asked for some instruments.

The next thing I knew, he opened the patient's abdomen with a knife right in the emergency room. "Jim, get some gloves on and help me," he said.

He cross-clamped the patient's aorta, and we moved to the operating room with our hands in this man's abdomen. We poured fluids and blood into him and started to get a faint pulse and blood pressure back.

The surgeon knew a vascular surgeon at the University of Wisconsin. He asked a nurse to notify the vascular surgery service of the event and made suggestions on equipment to bring up on a helicopter.

Helicopter transport was just getting started with the emergency transfer of patients. In the meantime, we each took turns leaving the patient to go scrub in with sterile technique while the other kept the aorta clamp securely in place.

Within the hour, I heard a helicopter land outside the hospital as we continued to work on the patient. In walked the University Hospital team, including a vascular surgeon. By now, we had obtained a pulse and a faint blood pressure. I scrubbed out and let the general surgeon and the University Hospital vascular surgeon complete the operation.

The patient left our hospital with a blood pressure and a pulse, although still not breathing on his own. He later in the week died at the University Hospital, unfortunately.

We had tried our best with the resources available. That patient might have lived had he had his collapse in the University Hospital lobby instead of ours.

When I had called the University Hospital to check on the patient, some of the questions the resident physicians asked me about the case were downright hurtful:

"Why don't you have a vascular surgeon on staff?"

"What kind of a hospital do you have up there?"

"How can you stand practicing at a Band-Aid station?"

Since those times, interns and residents don't ask these types of questions anymore. I attribute this to the fact that students now do some of their school rotations onsite in rural communities as part of their curriculum. They are also coached by their faculty not to say these things anymore.

I learned through the years to ignore these comments. A rural hospital will never equal the facilities of a larger urban hospital, but that is not an excuse to close rural hospitals. I knew that without our smaller hospital staff, people living in these areas would have no chance at all.

Several weeks later, I saw my last appointment of the day listed as "Family Conference." I was puzzled about this since, usually, I scheduled these types of conferences myself. They typically were used to cover a complex issue where we might need more time.

As I opened the exam room, I confronted two men and a woman probably in their forties. I introduced myself with a smile, extending my hand to everyone.

"Hello, I am Dr. Damos. You are the last appointment of the day, so we have plenty of time to talk about your concerns. What can I do for you?"

One of the men said, "We won't take long, Doc. We are the children of the man you attempted to save who ruptured an abdominal aortic aneurysm about a month ago. We wanted to come in and tell you how much we appreciated your efforts at trying to save our father's life. He was a wonderful man having farmed on the same farm for over fifty years. We are going to miss him a lot. We know you did everything you could, and we wanted to thank you."

Each of them stood up to shake my hand again.

"You know, I didn't know your father, but I wish I had. It is obvious your father participated in the raising of a wonderful family. I am certain it would have been a privilege for me to know him. I also want to thank you for coming here today. I can't emphasize enough to you how much this means to me."

Again, I thought to myself, so much for the myth about stubborn, narrow-minded, hard-to-get-along-with rural folks.

Another emergency occurred one winter in the middle of a snowstorm. On call, I visited the ER before I made the drive home in the snow.

Suddenly, a farmer comes in shouting and waving his hands wildly. "Help, help, my wife collapsed at home and is unconscious. She's in the back of my truck right outside."

Rather than wait for an ambulance to arrive at his farm, located far out in the country on snow-ridden roads, he had laid her in the back of his truck and rushed to the hospital.

We ran out with a stretcher. Initially, we were unable to find the patient, until we realized she was under the snow piled up in the bed of his vehicle. We brushed her off, placed her on the stretcher and rushed her into the emergency room.

On hooking her up to a cardiac monitor, we noted she had a very rapid pulse (tachycardia). The monitor complexes appeared regular and narrow. Since she was unstable, unconscious and with only faint blood pressure, we started an IV, gave her oxygen, and began to warm her aggressively. After getting her out of wet clothing, drying her off, and getting her into a hospital gown, I decided to electro-cardiovert (shock) her heart into a normal rhythm. This approach worked. She was admitted to our intensive care unit and recovered.

I am sure her ride in the snow in the bed of the truck, thus being cold and hypothermic, helped this patient, as hypothermia protects vital organs.

She later saw a cardiologist, who diagnosed her arrhythmia as the result of a defective electrical pathway in the heart. Her cardiac rhythm was then controlled with medication; although today cardiology has the tools to attempt an ablation of the alternative electrical path if needed.

Another emergency occurred one night when I was on call. A farmer had been plowing his field and was on the side of a hill when his tractor rolled on him. He arrived with what looked like a fractured and dislocated elbow. The pointed part of his elbow (called the olecranon) was displaced way backward and swollen, causing him a lot of pain.

As I went through my primary survey, taking an AMPLE history (**A**llergies, **M**edications, **P**ast History, **L**ast meal, **E**vents surrounding his injury), I noted his affected hand was very pale and cold. He had no pulse on his wrist. His x-rays showed a dislocation-fracture to his elbow.

Brachial artery injuries from elbow dislocations are uncommon, but they may lead to terrible consequences if not dealt with urgently. The brachial artery is the major artery that supplies the arm. With a dislocated elbow, this vessel is compromised. Often it is just kinked, cutting off blood supply to the rest of the extremity. Relocating the dislocation is essential and should be done as soon as possible.

I immediately called our orthopedist on call. At that time, we only had one orthopedist, who took county-wide call for several hospitals. When I reached him, he was in surgery at another hospital.

I informed him of the situation and will never forget his advice to me: "*Put the mustard to it, Jimbo.* You have to relocate the posterior dislocated elbow to improve circulation in his arm."

I called in our nurse anesthetist, and we took the patient to the operating room right away. The patient had not eaten since lunch, so he was sedated, and I pulled his elbow back into place. It made a sound like walking in quicksand as you pick your foot up.

Immediately, the color in his hand improved, and his hand became warm.

I placed his elbow in a posterior splint and sling, and we admitted him to the hospital for further pain control. Our orthopedist came over within a few hours to see the patient. He took the patient back to surgery as there was a fracture that needed fixing. He applauded me for the work I had done, which made my day.

Again, I wondered what would have happened if a primary care physician and a rural hospital had not been available in this case.

Chapter 12

A Major Family Crisis

IN THE MID-1980S, I HAD A SIZEABLE AND rewarding rural practice. I was busy during the day and on night call every fourth to fifth night. When not on call, I sometimes went in to help my partners if there was a need in the intensive care unit, obstetrics, or the emergency room. My partners did the same for me, as most rural doctors did. We learned a lot, developed medical experience, and had the gratifying experience knowing we were needed.

One evening, I returned home after a day of seeing patients at the office. Linda said, "Jim, Jenny has had too many unexplained fevers over the past few months. Repeated doctor visits are frustrating and exhausting. It seems like she's sick too much. What do you think is going on?"

Over the past several months, our five-year-old Jenny's fevers would last four to five days and then spontaneously resolve without any explanation. She was seen in the clinic, and her blood testing and urinalysis were always normal.

"Linda, I think your concern is valid. I will talk with Dr. Bob at the clinic to see what he thinks about these recurrent fevers. I agree something is not right."

Before supper one night, I was playing with my two children. We played a game called "stand on hands" where I lay on my back, they stood on the palms of my hands, and I lifted them into a standing position. I then lowered them back down or caught them. As I played with Jenny, I felt a mass in her abdomen. I quickly turned her over and placed her on her back on the floor. In her right flank, there appeared to be an immobile mass. I flashed back to the child I saw as an urgent care work-in patient with a similar abdominal mass; this child, it turned out, had advanced cancer and later died.

I called my physician partner, Dr. Bob. "Bob, I hate to bother you this evening, but I am worried. I was playing with the kids, and I think I can feel an abdominal mass in Jenny's abdomen."

"Jim, it is likely some fecal matter that has not moved through the colon yet," he replied. "Why don't you recheck her in the morning and if it is still there, I will be happy to work her into my schedule tomorrow. Calm down, get some sleep, and see how she is in the morning. Let me know tomorrow if you are still concerned."

The next morning, I got up early to check Jenny. I had not slept well. I felt this was a mass and not stool. The abnormality was still present, and I panicked, my worst fear realized.

As promised, Dr. Bob worked Jenny into his schedule. An x-ray showed a mass in the right flank. Our hearts sank. Life was about to change significantly for our family.

Just like I had done with other children in my practice, Dr. Bob referred us to a pediatric surgeon and a pediatric oncologist in Madison. Further testing revealed a large mass in Jenny's right kidney, requiring surgery.

We alerted friends and family. Within hours, we had plenty of support. Our parents arrived; my mother was especially worried. Jenny was her pride and joy. Linda's parents were also stricken with grief as they loved Jenny so much and had participated in babysitting. They had cared for Jenny on several occasions when Linda and I had taken some needed husband-wife time away.

Our lives had changed dramatically in a matter of hours. Our two-year-old son, Tim, headed off with family members while Linda and I took up residence at the hospital. It seemed as if all of Reedsburg had been alerted. The cards began to pour in as did phone calls offering support. Many of my patients were distressed at the news.

The next morning, the pediatric surgeon visited with us before the operation. To me, he appeared emotionless and too blunt. He maintained weak eye contact, talked in a monotone, and cut off conversation quickly. I assumed it was because he was overly busy, especially since he was considered an excellent pediatric surgeon. He would later become a family friend.

Jenny was to go into the operating room at 7:30 a.m. A nurse came into our hospital room at seven. She said, "Unfortunately, there has been a severe auto accident.

All the operating rooms are currently dealing with the victims. Jenny's surgery has been postponed until further notice. I am sorry, but we will keep you up to date with any changes."

We understood priorities, but the delay was painful. As we waited, all kinds of things went through my head.

Am I the cause of her getting possible cancer? Was I carrying a gene? Did my working with lead-based paint by painting street signs during a summer job or working with chemicals cleaning rugs cause this? Did Linda have a gene that she transmitted? Could we have caught this earlier? Why would God do this to us? We have tried our best to live a moral, ethical, humanitarian life.

It is common to blame oneself or scapegoat others when faced with a severe and life-threatening disease.

Finally, at eleven a.m., they come to get our daughter. "You can carry Jenny to the operating room," the nurse said to me.

Scared, Jenny cried. "Daddy, Daddy don't leave me. Daddy, Daddy, please, I don't want to go here. Daddy, Daddy." She had a tight, white-knuckle hug around my neck and a terrified look on her face as I tried to hand her to the staff at the entrance to the operating room. It was heartbreaking, but I had to be strong, in control, and supportive. It took all I could muster to remain composed.

"I will be right outside honey. You are going to take a nap for a few hours. I want you to rest and think of us having fun when you wake up. Just like we do at home when we play stand on hands or you and Tim dance to the musical *Cats*." Trying to hold back tears, I felt my eyes welling up.

This experience helped me understand even more what my patients go through. I turned Jenny over to the operating room staff. I waved goodbye to her and blew her a kiss, wondering if I would see her ever again.

A nun from the hospital recognized my agony and sat with me during Jenny's operation. We prayed together, and she never left my side the entire afternoon. When I asked her why God would do this to anyone, she said, "I don't know why this happened to you. God works in mysterious ways." A more honest and believable answer than, "You have been chosen for growth, or your family will be stronger later."

This nun provided such comfort to Linda and me in our time of need.

Six hours later, the pediatric surgeon visited us in the waiting room. "The mass has been removed, as has Jenny's right kidney," he reported. "The mass was large, weighing about four pounds. It appeared to extend into the renal vein exiting the kidney. There did not seem to be any spread elsewhere."

The pathology report followed in a few days. The pediatric oncologist, Dr. Paul, summoned Linda and me to a conference room. My mother asked me to be at the conference as well. Dr. Paul and his nurse practitioner, Charlotte, ran this meeting expertly and with kindness. It was apparent he was skilled at doing this.

He started with introductions. In an empathic way, he said, "I know you have all been through a lot the past few days. This is never easy. I have the pathology report. I was initially concerned this may be neuroblastoma which is not good. Instead, this is what is called a Wilms tumor. It has favorable histology and is what we call stage II. This is treatable."

I asked, "What treatment is recommended? How treatable?"

He responded, "We can enter Jenny into a research trial. Four different treatment regimens are being studied right now. She will be randomized to one of the four treatment regimens which include various combinations of chemotherapy including Actinomycin D, Vincristine, and Adriamycin, with or without radiation."

I was very uncomfortable with my daughter being "randomized" to a regimen where the outcome was currently unknown. What if she ended up on the worst of the four regimens?

Dr. Paul and his nurse practitioner skillfully answered everyone's questions, taking the needed time to make us all feel heard. The conference ended after I said I would like to think about the randomization issue.

Linda stayed at the hospital that night. There were rooms at the hospital where parents could sleep and be with their child right down the hall. The nursing staff was excellent at accommodating parents who had a sick child admitted.

Back in Reedsburg, I spent most of the night in our hospital library reading about Wilms tumor and the four regimens being studied. At about five a.m., one of our excellent nurses came in, spoke with me in an empathic kind manner and urged me to go home and get some sleep. I came away, however, with an opinion on what regimen I felt might be the best for Jenny. I preferred Jenny to be on Actinomycin D, Vincristine, and radiation following her surgery. Adriamycin had effects on the heart that scared me. The pediatric oncologist was flexible and agreed to this regimen. Jenny would not be randomized but instead placed on one of the four regimens I had read about which seemed to be the most successful to date.

In the following days, Linda and I took turns staying with our daughter in the pediatric intensive care unit. We stayed at the hospital while family, neighbors, and friends stayed with our son, Tim. The hospital accommodated all parents who had sick children that were admitted. We did not seek status for physicians and their families.

One night on my turn to stay with Jenny in the intensive care unit, Linda retired to the hospital room to sleep. At two a.m., as I lightly slept off and on in a chair next to Jenny's hospital bed, I stared at our daughter, wondering what would happen. She had a tube in her nose going down to her stomach. She was wearing oxygen, had an IV hooked up to her arm, a catheter in her bladder, a blood pressure cuff on her left arm and heart monitor wires on her chest.

Suddenly she woke up and in a very soft voice said, "Daddy, daddy, come here."

I got up out of my chair and leaned down to hear what she had to say. Placing my ear near her mouth, I said, "What do you need, honey?"

In a whisper, she said, "Daddy, you don't look so good. You better go home and get some sleep."

There she was, the one hooked up to all the tubes and monitors, and she had concern for me.

❧

Jenny recovered from her surgery and returned home, only to develop a fever a few days after discharge. She ended up back in the hospital with a suspected pelvic abscess. After more tests and several days of intravenous antibiotics, no further surgery was necessary.

After recovering from the second hospital admission, Jenny went for her radiation at the University of Wisconsin Hospital. She needed fifteen months of chemotherapy with intravenous actinomycin D and vincristine given every month for five days out of the month.

Once Jenny's chemotherapy schedule stabilized, I returned to work, but I lightened my patient schedule. My partners were excellent at giving me the time I needed when I needed it.

My physician partner and our family physician, Dr. Bob, had delivered Jenny into this world. He administered her chemotherapy over the next fifteen months under the guidance of Dr. Paul, the pediatric oncologist. We lived an hour away from the specialty center; it was common practice in those days for the primary care physician to administer the chemotherapy, since the oncologist did not come to our small community. Driving to Madison for five days in a row each month for chemotherapy with a child in the car who might become nauseated on the way home was frowned upon.

Dr. Bob did an excellent job administering this chemotherapy by daily intravenous sticks into Jenny's hand or arm, without the use of today's skin-tunneled central venous catheters or Hickman or Groshong lines. These lines were not as prevalent then, and Jenny wanted to swim during the summer.

As I returned to work, I felt the stress of being in rural practice while having a child on cancer treatment. The burden of a busy rural medical practice, the trauma cases I dealt with in the emergency room, and the sometimes-erratic hours of maternity care began to wear on me.

The emotions parents go through during a childhood cancer are volatile. My mind ran rampant at night with thoughts that kept me lying awake.

Will she live?

I just heard her cough in her sleep. Is she getting pneumonia? This is her week on chemotherapy, and her immune system is suppressed.

She is losing her hair. She will look different from other kids. How will we handle possible bullying? Will her hair grow back the same as before?

Is she in any pain?

What if she gets sick and ends up in the hospital near death? How will we respond to hospice-type care for our child if it comes to that?

How is Linda holding up? She looks much stronger than I, but is she hiding her feelings?

I need to play with Tim more. I don't want him to feel neglected.

One night, I was sitting in the hospital maternity unit, following two women in labor. One was dilated to five centimeters and the other to seven centimeters. Both were experiencing intense contractions and moving along rapidly. I wondered if I would need to be in two places at once.

As I contemplated calling in one of my partners to help, the obstetric nurse handed me the phone. "Your wife is on the line."

"Jim, Jenny has a fever, and she's on chemotherapy this week. What should I do?" Linda asked me.

"Take her into the emergency room. I will meet you down there when these two women deliver," I said. "They are close. You can bring Tim with you or maybe call a neighbor to come over in case he wakes up."

Fortunately, both women delivered uneventfully back to back. I went down to the emergency room where I met Linda and Jenny. Her fever was low grade, and all her tests including lab and chest x-ray were normal. The ER doctor consulted with the on-call pediatric oncologist in Madison, and it was decided Jenny had a minor viral infection. She recovered without complications.

That night, however, I became serious about making a change in my life. Linda too felt increasingly stressed. Despite an outpouring of support from family, friends, neighbors, and community, childhood cancer is exceedingly stressful. Studies have shown that close to half the caregivers of a child with cancer experience severe strain. Quality of life is impaired, including sleep quality, diet, and exercise habits.

With me working as a physician, Linda was the primary caregiver. She had to deal with such challenges as nausea, vomiting, fever, crying, and giving the needed attention to Tim during the day. Many of our friends were kind, but gun shy about coming over and potentially giving Jenny an infection. Whereas we used to have fun with friends, it was now more of a sympathy visit when we were visited. It's difficult to comprehend these changing relationships until you go through it yourself.

I taught Advanced Cardiac Life Support in our rural county. I had noticed several medical journal articles authored by the University of Wisconsin Department of Family Medicine faculty physicians. One report by Dr. William Scheibel (University of Wisconsin faculty) and Dr. Susan Isensee (University of Wisconsin Verona Clinic family medicine resident) presented a case of multiple sclerosis. This well-written journal article made an impression on me.

In exploring the job offerings in the back of the journals, I noted a position open at the University of Wisconsin Department of Family Medicine. I thought I might apply for it. The call nights would be fewer with more physicians sharing call. With residents taking after-hours coverage with me, it would take away a lot of paperwork and inject the opportunity to teach into the equation, which I enjoyed. Finally, living in Madison, we would be closer to the oncology center in case of cancer recurrence. Perhaps it was time for a change.

As I thought about such a move, I felt scattered and paralyzed. I used to make quick decisions in the emergency room and maternity care center, but this was different.

Linda appeared much more level-headed, but the strain began to wear on her. She took Jenny in for most of her chemotherapy injections. She handled Jenny's chemotherapy side effects with expert, kind, motherly care. I often saw her speak in a soft, calm, reassuring voice when Jenny became ill and vomited after her injections. Linda kept me on track with the same encouraging, loving behavior. By all outward appearances, she was a rock; but I knew it wore on her.

The idea of leaving Reedsburg, Wisconsin, was very hard for us as we contemplated this decision. We had a lovely home, great friends, and a supportive extended family living within two to three hours of us. I had a thriving and bustling rural practice with good physician partners. However, we felt it necessary to leave for many reasons, mostly related to my burnout and Linda's increasing strain.

As we went through the process of listing our house, informing my partners of our plans, applying for a new job with the University of Wisconsin Department of Family Medicine, and looking for a new home, we had second thoughts.

I remember talking to a couple—old friends of ours since our medical school days in St. Louis. They had come to visit us from New York to offer their comfort and support. Dr. Bob Kottkamp was a professor of Education at Hofstra University; his wife, Ginny, was a nurse midwife working in Brooklyn. They advised us to weigh the pros and cons of a move.

We drew a line down the center of a piece of paper and listed the advantages and disadvantages of moving. We made the decision to leave, and Ginny and Bob advised us now to *destroy the alternatives*. This approach of making an informed decision and then killing the other options turned out to be the advice that helped us the most.

Chapter 13

A Difficult Decision

SAYING GOODBYE TO FRIENDS, CO-WORKERS, and patients ripped my heart out. The hospital staff put together an album of pictures of all the employees from various hospital departments, which I have retained to this day. One nurse made a beautiful wall clock for me with the letters RMH for Reedsburg Memorial Hospital, which still hangs in our home. Linda would miss our house on five acres with its beautiful garden as gardening was her primary hobby.

It was a good time in our family cycle to leave while our kids were still young. We did not send Jenny to kindergarten while she was on chemotherapy. She had not had chicken pox yet, and the chicken pox vaccine had not then been developed. I can't blame our friends for keeping their kids away from her. Chickenpox could kill a child on chemotherapy in the 1980s. We held her out of school the first year while on chemo. The Reedsburg School District supplied us with a homeschooling kindergarten teacher. I thought this was going above and beyond the call of duty to provide a home teacher for *kindergarten.* Remember the myth, "I hear the school systems out there are not as good?"

The second year, Jenny attended first grade in town after she completed her chemotherapy. We were concerned about whether to let her ride a school bus with older kids. It was hard enough for us to see our daughter as frail as she was, including her hair loss, just beginning to grow back. We worried about bullying or her being picked on during her school bus rides. The pediatric oncologist advised we treat her like any other child. He felt it was vital for her to learn how to socialize and live life like other little girls.

We were pleasantly surprised to see the kids on the school bus become protective of her, even the high school kids. I watched her get off the school bus one afternoon waving goodbye to all the kids waving back at her as she came running up the driveway, her school backpack almost tipping over her frail, skinny body.

We were still not out of the woods with her follow-up for recurrent cancer, but things at least were more stable, making a move possible.

On the office front, many of my patients came in to say goodbye after we publicly announced our decision to leave. We reminisced about hospitalizations, obstetric deliveries, home visits, and surgeries we'd gone through during my ten years.

One of my ten-year patients was a man I will call Hank, a very polite man whose wife I also followed. Despite her many chronic illnesses, his wife was one of the most positive people I've ever met. She never complained about anything and kept a smile on her face ninety percent of the time. I had admitted her to the hospital on numerous occasions over my ten years in Reedsburg, because of complications from these chronic illnesses. Hank was supportive of his wife but had his own set of neurologic problems. It seemed he could not feel anything in his left arm, which was weak and did not function well. Hank had visited numerous neurologists at the University Hospital and through the VA system with no diagnosis made. He had emphasized to me often during his office visits that he was a veteran of World War II.

Hank's last visit with me came on a Monday, the first patient of the day. He brought his wife in with him as they wanted to say goodbye and thank me for the care I had given them over the years. Hank was the more emotional of the two that day.

As we got into the visit, tears began to stream down his face as he looked down at the floor.

I thought, wow, it can't be this emotional to leave your doctor.

As I was ready to go and say goodbye, Hank said, "Please wait a minute. I want to tell you something I have never told anyone."

I paused and again sat down. Hank appeared to be almost shaking now while he cried. *Something else is going on here*. His wife was quite attentive. Her usual smile had disappeared.

"You remember. Doc, I was in World War II, and I am a veteran. War was not my thing. I am a nonviolent person. In fact, during battle, I often shot over the heads of the enemy. I couldn't bear to kill another human being, thinking they had a mom and dad, brothers and sisters; you know, just like us."

I remained silent but attentive as he continued, "One night, Doc, we were in a firefight. My squad members noticed I was shooting high. They figured out what I was doing."

He continued. "When the firefight was over, the guys confronted me and accused me of shooting over the heads of people, which I denied. To put me on the spot, they brought in a captured enemy soldier and placed him in front of me. He looked to be about eighteen years old. They told me to 'shoot him in the head and prove I was fighting for America.'"

Hank's voice went up an octave as the tears flowed. "Doc, I have never told anyone this. That enemy soldier began to cry and plead with me not to shoot. The squad cheered for me to pull the trigger. I felt threatened by my own fellow soldiers that night. Finally, I shot him in the forehead and killed him. It was a matter of survival for me. I sacrificed this young man to save myself. I cannot forgive myself for what I did. I am left-handed and held the gun in my left hand. I haven't felt anything in my left arm since. It doesn't function well."

Hank had what in psychological terms is a conversion reaction. Since I was now leaving town, he felt compelled to confess to someone he trusted. His wife was shocked, as Hank apparently had spared her this story through the years.

I said, "Hank, this was not your fault. You were in a difficult situation. Anyone would have considered what you faced that night as the ultimate challenge. War is awful. Hank, I do respect those who wear the uniform and serve our country. You did what you had to do that night to survive. It was not your fault."

I suggested he consider seeing a mental health therapist, and his wife promised she would try to get him to follow through.

I felt a great privilege talking to the patients who came to see me that day. Almost every one of them had their own stories to tell me during these reminiscence sessions, but I felt none would match what Hank had confided in me.

Photos

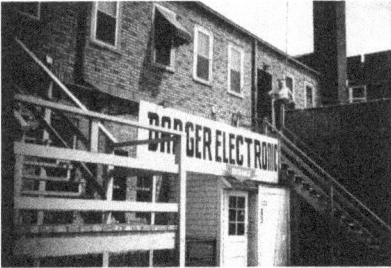

Backdoor of Dr. Damos' Waukegan home where his extended family and he lived. His apartment was at the top of the stairs to the left. His uncle is standing on the steps of his family's apartment.

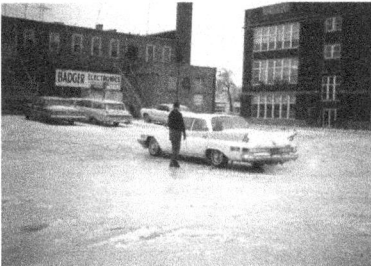

Back parking lot of Dr. Damos' Waukegan home with the high school to the right. A large parking lot was the "back yard" growing up.

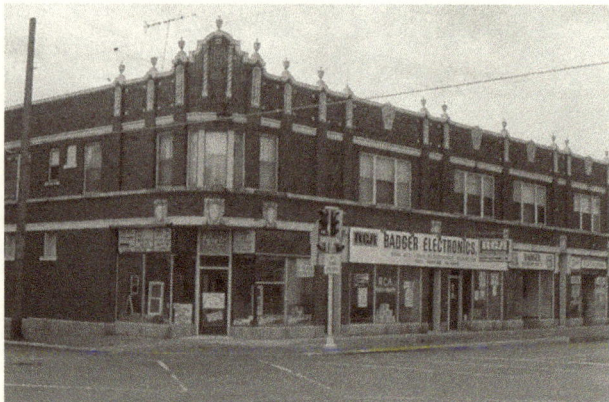

Front of Dr. Damos' Waukegan home. His family living room is the second set of triple windows from the right. The family restaurant (W' Shop) is on the corner. The high school is across the street to the left out of the picture.

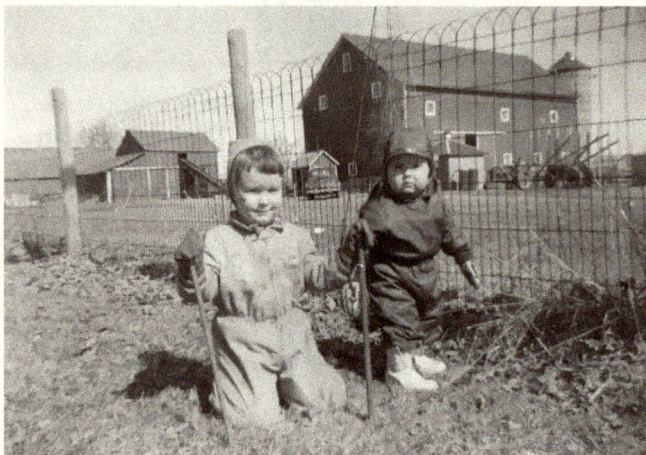

Linda Damos and her brother on their dairy farm. Her dad in those years plowed his fields with horses.

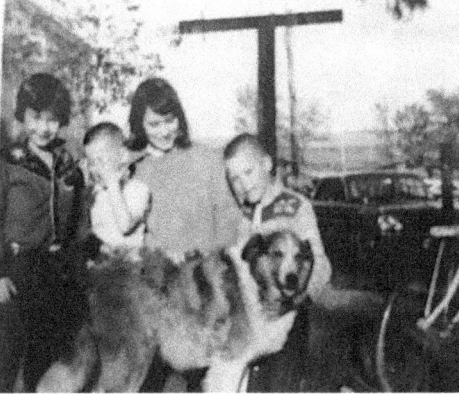

Linda in the center during her college years with her two brothers (Tom, Dave), her sister (Margaret) and their Collie dog.

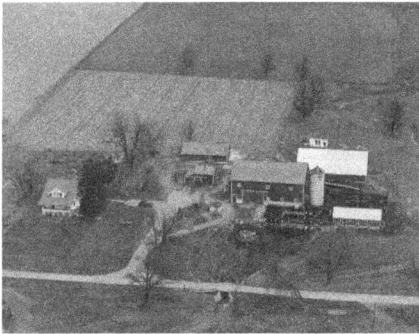

Aerial view of Linda's farm in the 1950s

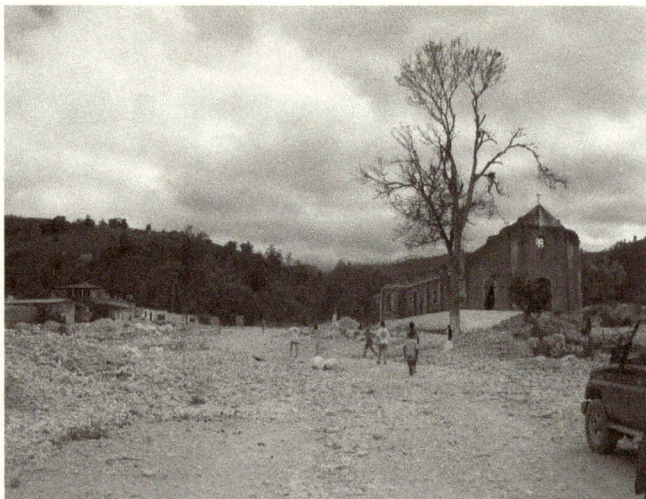

The road to Thiotte, Haiti

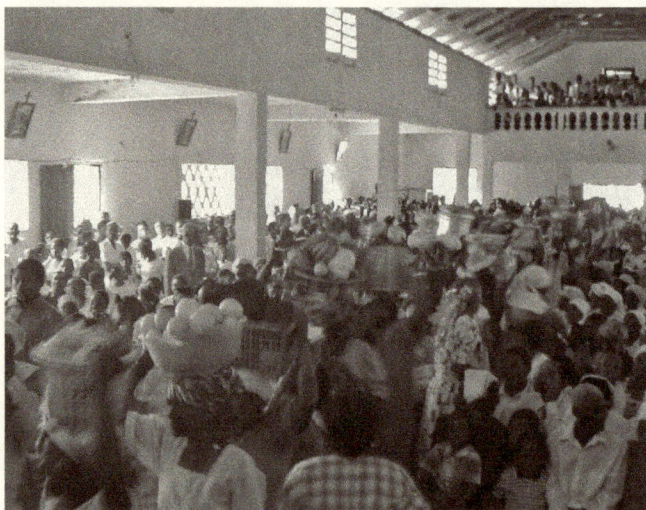

Haitians dancing up the aisle with gifts to the music of a children's choir. This was a church service held at the beginning of the Haiti medical mission.

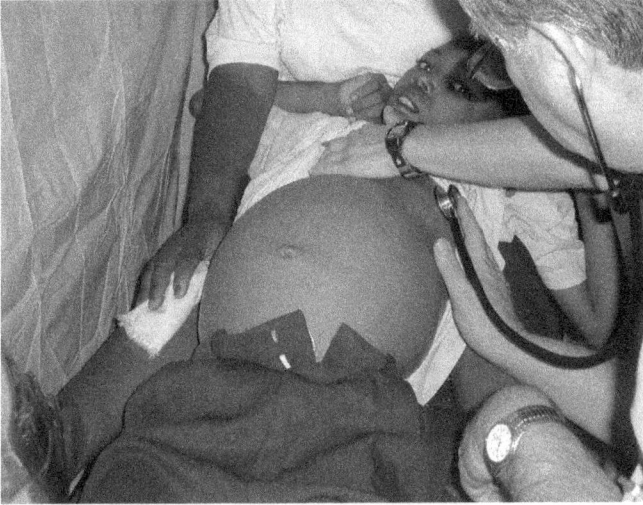

Dr. Damos examining a boy with a large belly who couldn't efficiently inhale. The child had mitral valve stenosis with a heart murmur and congestive heart failure. Fluid fills this boy's abdomen. This is called ascites. He couldn't breathe well. A diuretic was administered and he began to excrete water and breathe easier.

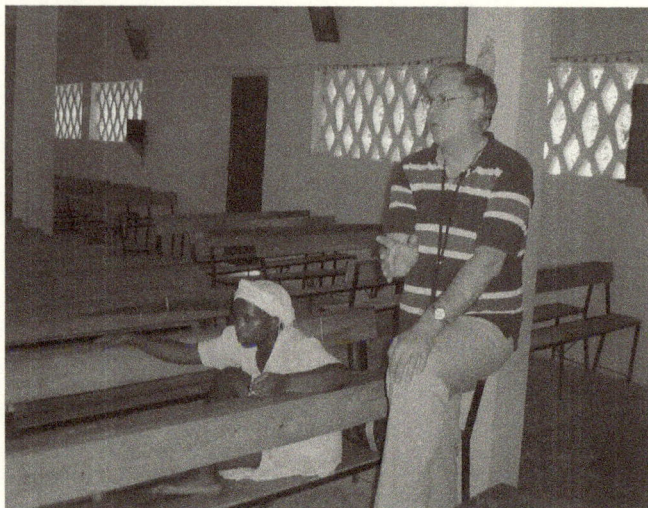

Dr. Damos with a teenager who had tetanus (lockjaw). She had stepped on a nail.

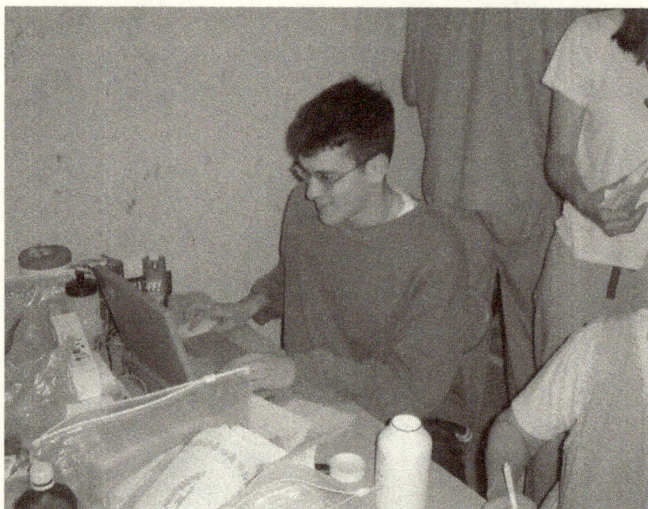

Tim Damos working creating medical records for Haitians.

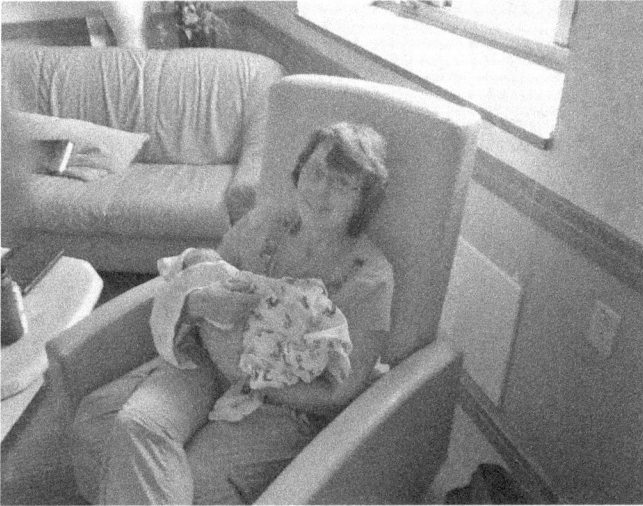

Grandchild Aleyna born on Linda's birthday 2012. What a gift from daughter, Jenny.

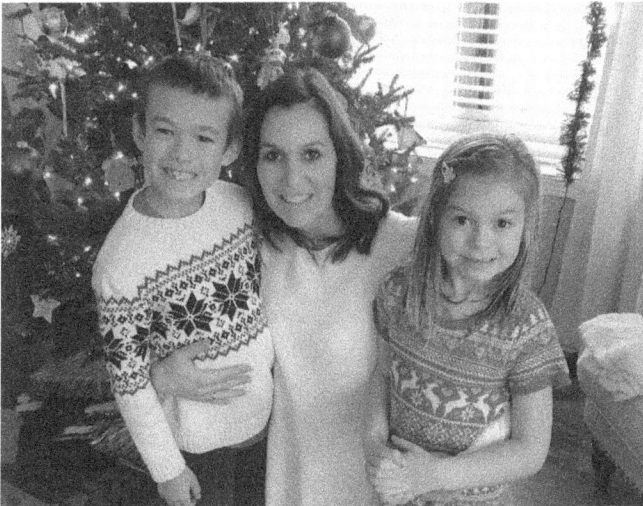

Jenny and her children, Kyan and Aleyna. Jenny is now an elementary school psychologist.

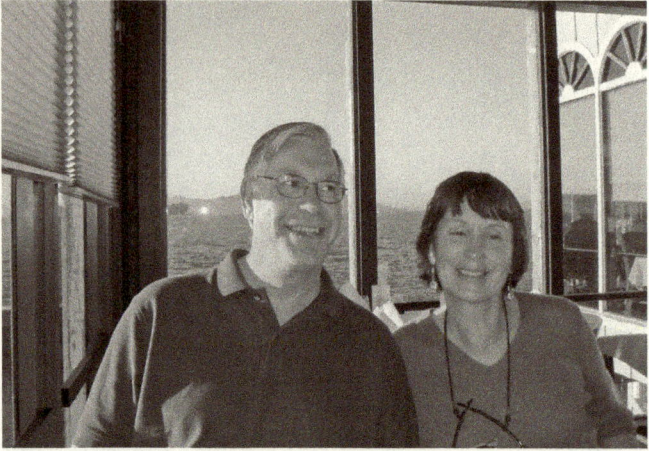
Jim and Linda in San Francisco at a medical conference.

Academics and Teaching

Chapter 14

The Move and Rebounding

W E HAD A BIT MORE MONEY FOR THIS MOVE, despite our continuing medical school loans, and hired a mover to move us to the Madison, Wisconsin area. Linda and I shopped for homes but saw nothing that excited us. We had sold our Reedsburg home right away despite the higher interest rates.

One evening, Linda returned home after spending the day house-hunting. "Jim, I found a corner lot in a subdivision called Ravenoaks in Oregon, Wisconsin just a few miles south of Madison. Would you ever consider us building a home?"

I replied, "I guess I never thought about it. We will have to rent while the house is built. Do you have a plan in mind?"

She replied excitedly, "As a matter of fact, I have been searching plans and have a few in mind. I can look for an apartment to rent for a few months. By the way, I met a teacher while looking at this corner lot today. She was getting her mail and lives across the street from the lot. I stopped to chat with her and ask about the neighborhood."

"And . . . ?"

"What a pleasant person. She loves the neighbor-hood, and I bet she would be a great neighbor. I chatted with her for about thirty minutes. Her name is Kay."

This little chat turned out to be a rewarding one-to-one for our family's recovery. Kay Johnston and Linda became the best of friends. The Johnston and Damos families to this day do things together and support each other through whatever life throws at us, even though distance has become a small factor.

We searched out a builder, and Linda gladly embarked on her positive and forward-looking project.

We rented an apartment in a suburb. The kids enrolled in school, and Linda drove them to and from school every day (about ten miles to and from our temporary apartment). I started my new job at the University of Wisconsin.

Every evening, Linda reported on the development of the house-building project. We couldn't wait for it to be completed for two reasons. First, we were novices at building a home. We had fun seeing it go up little by little and were anxious to move in. Second, we had bites, yes bites.

One evening after dinner, I saw Linda, Jenny, Tim, and our dog Pepper all scratching at once. "Why is everyone scratching?" I said.

I checked the kids. They had what looked like small red bumps below their knees. Each little red bump had a red halo around it. On Jenny, the bites appeared in groups of three or four and on Tim, they looked like a straight line starting at the ankle and moving up the leg. These were flea bites. I called a professional pest control service and gave some hydrocortisone cream to everyone to use on the itches. We washed and powdered the dog with flea treatment.

After four months, our house was built, and we moved in. Ravenoaks was a remarkable neighborhood, just what we needed after so many stressful days in our past.

We met another physician who lived down the street from us, a pediatric allergist, Dr. Brent Kooistra, an excellent doctor, and a great neighbor. Our son, Tim, and his son, Scott, became close friends. They watched movies together, played basketball, and generally hung out together at one or the other's house. Scott later became a weightlifter and took an interest in football. He went on to play college football at North Carolina State and then played in the NFL with the Cincinnati Bengals and Minnesota Vikings as a tackle. He was rough on the field but one of the kindest, gentlest people ever when not wearing football equipment.

Jenny was now off cancer treatment, and she was being followed every six months for recurrence of cancer. Her hair had come back more beautiful than ever, and she had a healthy look about her again. Her follow-up to date had been favorable.

Kay's husband, Dave, and I became friends. Dave sold insurance and managed investments. He arranged an annual fishing trip to Canada for a group of guys, which I enjoyed being part of.

Our Ravenoaks neighborhood was a great place to raise a family. On Halloween, the whole community participated in the festivities. People visited make-shift graveyards built on front lawns; one of the family garages was made into a "house of horror;" and children wandered around the neighborhood trick-or-treating during the evening. Our pediatric allergist friend, Dr. Brent, sat in a field and howled through a vacuum cleaner hose to scare people.

We spent many an evening combining dinners for an outdoor feast with neighborhood friends or going out for Friday night fish fry (a Wisconsin tradition). Dave and Kay's kids across the street became close friends with our children. Jenny developed a friendship with Nikki Johnston, and they remain just like sisters to this day. Our family enjoyed fun times with new friends.

Linda found a position with the University of Wisconsin Department of Environmental Toxicology, studying the effects of pollution on fish in the Great Lakes. She developed relationships at work and felt satisfied with her scientific job and fellow staff.

I worked as an assistant professor at the University of Wisconsin Department of Family Medicine. The UW–Madison physician training program had forty-two residents distributed at four residency clinics throughout the Madison area. Approximately thirty family physician faculty members along with a great staff of nurse practitioners, physician assistants, nurses, and clerical staff provided primary care. Each clinic had its own complement of first-, second-, and third-year resident physicians in training. Medical students rotated through our sites on their primary care rotations. Mental health therapists were based at each clinic to provide on-site counseling. Pharmacist faculty taught at each location to help the residents scrutinize patient medication lists. There were in-house x-ray and lab at each clinic, and a visiting physical therapist from the University Hospital came out weekly. This was the ideal primary care clinic. It was one-stop primary care shopping for the patient. I met some great people and felt like a real physician quarterback managing the team for the patient, who was the coach.

My partners at our teaching clinic supported me as the newcomer. They were competent physicians and became great friends. Dr. Bill Scheibel (who had written the journal article on multiple sclerosis with Dr. Susan Isensee that impressed me) and his wife, Pam (a pediatric nurse practitioner and professor on the faculty at the University of Wisconsin School of Nursing), became lifelong friends. Dr. Scheibel was an excellent physician. I respected his knowledge of primary care and his positive approach to life.

Another clinic faculty physician who helped me adapt was Dr. John Beasley, a very welcoming person who became one of my mentors into academics. A veteran of the department, he had been around the block in academics locally, regionally, and nationally.

I found the rest of the clinic staff to be terrific people. They welcomed me with open arms and showed me the ropes. I felt like this would be a great place to work.

Our residency training clinic was a small building with creaking floors and a winding staircase that went downstairs to the business offices. We were pretty much jammed tightly together, sharing office space and rotating exam rooms. Despite our overcrowding, we seemed to have a great time together seeing our patients and navigating the day.

Our patient clientele was diverse. We saw young professionals, people working at the university, and farm families who traveled to see us from the west side of the state. There was a significant senior population with two local nursing homes that we attended. I completed extra training in geriatrics, passed my Certificate of Added Qualifications in Geriatrics, and began teaching geriatrics in the residency. I became the medical director of two local nursing homes in the Madison area. I saw patients part-time and taught physical diagnosis at the medical school. I found this variety of tasks stimulating and rewarding.

My first year of academics was under development. I missed the challenge in my old job in rural practice, where you often had to think outside the box because of the lack of readily available on-site specialty backup. However, I gained teaching skills in Madison interacting with some of the sharpest residents in the nation who had come to our University of Wisconsin family medicine residency. As I taught physical diagnosis at the medical school and worked with the resident physicians in training, I often told stories about

the fascinating cases I had encountered in rural practice. My small-town practice helped me immensely in
teaching.

❧

June 1988, the evening of the resident graduation banquet. The residents from the four clinics came together
to celebrate their completion of three years of residency
training. The dinner launched them into their careers.
I was disappointed about being on call the night of my
first graduation banquet with the residency, probably a
rite of passage for those new on the faculty. Linda and I
still planned to attend the dinner, realizing I might get
called out. Residents on call might call me with questions or see a hospital patient. I wore a beeper and carried the clinic's large mobile phone, almost the size of a
small football in 1988.

The dinner had around one hundred people in attendance, including faculty, staff, residents, and their family members. During the meal, my beeper went off. I
called the number which turned out to be the emergency room. A nurse summoned the resident physician
to the phone to talk with me.

"Dr. Damos, I have a child here who fell on his out-
stretched hand while riding a bike. His wrist is bruised
and swollen. I have ordered an x-ray," the resident
reported.

"I'll be right there. I am about fifteen minutes away,"
I replied. I notified Linda I was leaving. Dr. Scheibel

said he and Pam could give Linda a ride home if I didn't get back in time.

When I arrived at the emergency room, the resident and I reviewed this child's x-ray.

"What do you see?" I challenged the resident's x-ray interpretation.

"Well, I see a fracture of his radius."

"Good job," I said. "And how do you want to treat this little guy?"

The resident physician came up with a proper treatment plan, as did most of the residents and interns in this program. The UW Family Medicine program attracted top-notch talent. It turned out this child had a minor non-displaced distal radial buckle (wrist) fracture, which is a small fracture. We placed him in a splint with instructions on care and follow-up. I had time to return to the banquet.

As I entered the banquet room, everyone turned around, stood up and clapped. Dumbfounded, I turned around to see what was going on behind me. I hadn't taught fracture care to the resident physician on call that well to earn a standing ovation.

I heard the announcement: "Dr. Damos, you have earned the distinct honor of winning the Baldwin E. Lloyd Teacher of the Year award this year, voted on by the residents and interns in the program."

What an honor for me. I flashed back to that night a few years ago on call in Reedsburg when there were two women in labor in the middle of the night, and Linda called to tell me Jenny was on chemotherapy and had a fever. I contrast the sinking feeling I felt that night with this honor of being voted teacher of the year.

On returning home that night Linda and I revisited our conflicting feelings about leaving Reedsburg. "Any second thoughts now," Linda said to me. We always had second thoughts about whether we had made the right decision.

"Nope, I think we made the right decision," I replied. "Besides, Jenny is doing so well now. Her follow-up is going well, and all tests to date have been normal. She has developed a circle of friends and is doing well in school. She is smiling a lot, and no longer has the appearance of a frail, thin, sick little child."

Tim was also fine. He made friends, did well in school, and enjoyed our neighborhood. Life was good.

Chapter 15

Perceived Differences— Rural vs. Urban

BEING ON STAFF AS AN ASSISTANT PROFESSOR of family medicine at the University of Wisconsin–Madison was a job entirely different from my former rural practice.

My Reedsburg practice day started at seven or eight in the morning with hospital rounds. I walked into my rural hospital and received a warm greeting from the staff at the nurse's station. Someone would hand me a cup of coffee and point toward the donuts.

A nurse would approach me with a cart that had my patient charts on it. She then made rounds with me and shared patient data and observations by the nursing staff. I saw an average of three to five, sometimes up to ten, patients in the hospital before going to the clinic. If the surgeon asked me for help with a surgical case, I adjusted my clinic schedule accordingly. By ten a.m., I saw patients for the rest of the day in my office at the clinic.

For an emergency, or if I had a baby to deliver, it took a five-minute walk through a tunnel that connected the clinic with the hospital. My after-hours call was every fourth or fifth night. There was no rush hour traffic to deal with on the way to the hospital, no parking garages to navigate, and the entire staff at the hospital knew each other. Cardiac arrests and other emergencies were conducted efficiently and competently in the small town because staff members were familiar with each other and felt comfortable working together during a crisis. Most were trained in basic and advanced cardiac life support and effectively used the protocols.

I found academics and urban medicine an entirely different type of practice. After-hours call ranged every tenth to fourteenth night; better lifestyle, but less challenging. Four residency clinics were located throughout Madison. We admitted medical and pediatric patients to the university hospital and to one of the private hospitals. We delivered obstetric patients at two of the private hospitals. Things could get chaotic when taking clinic after-hours calls; admitting patients to more than one hospital meant driving back and forth.

Driving up to the hospital meant engaging with traffic on the expressways and navigating a tiered parking garage before entering the hospital. Once inside, the hospital staff didn't know me that well, so it was common for a nurse to ask me if I was a family member or a minister. The hospital specialty floors felt tribal if you weren't part of the specialty of that floor.

To avoid daytime hospital care chaos in my academic job, we ran inpatient hospital teaching services at two hospitals. One faculty member would supervise a team of resident physicians for two weeks, once in the fall and once again in the spring. This reduced my hospital practice of medicine from daily hospital rounds in Reedsburg to four weeks per year in Madison. However, these four weeks were an intense hospital patient care experience. Our teaching service admitted patients from any of the four residency clinics. The patients were unfamiliar to the team and to the faculty member. Their clinic doctor rarely visited them in the hospital. This was a breakdown of continuity of care but educational for the learners who challenged the faculty on service.

Pregnant patients from any of the four residency clinics were admitted to one of two private hospitals; entirely different than small-town practice.

This patient care system was complicated and challenging. I noted the other faculty physicians also felt challenged with the operation of this care system. This patient care structure was dictated by geography, hospital/HMO affiliations, and student education. The call and coverage system came up as an issue often at faculty meetings. Patient handoffs, call trades, hospital coverage, and skill levels and interests of faculty members were topics of discussion. I am not saying this care system was wrong, just different than what I had been used to.

I found the patient clientele slightly different compared to my former small-town medical practice. Many factors influenced this rural/urban patient cultural difference. Because specialty physicians are more accessible to the urban population, urban patients requested referrals more often, consequently making the cost of healthcare higher.

I remember seeing a high school basketball player one afternoon in the clinic. He came in with a sprained ankle. His father accompanied him.

"Hello, I'm Doctor Damos. Nice to meet you both. I understand we have an injured basketball player here," I said. "Did your injury occur during a slam dunk? You look like you could do one of those."

Smiling, his father said, "No, it wasn't a dunk. He was running down court during a game when his ankle gave out. He came off the court limping. I think he needs an x-ray and referral to sports medicine. Even though he's only a sophomore, I think he has a future in NCAA Division I basketball. He is pretty good."

There is a questionnaire we use in primary care called the Ottawa Ankle Rules that has five questions. The answers to these questions help us decide whether an x-ray is warranted or not. The five questions are as follows:

1. Could the patient bear weight and take four steps immediately after the injury?

   a. He answered, "Yes, but it hurt."

2. Is there bony tenderness over the outer portion of the ankle (the lateral malleolus)?

   a. When I examined him, he had no bony tenderness there.

3. Is there bony tenderness over the inner part of the ankle (medial malleolus)

   a. He had no bony soreness over the inner part of the ankle.

4. Is there pain over the outer part of the foot (base of the 5th metatarsal)

   a. He had no tenderness over the outer part of the foot.

5. Is there pain on the inner foot (over the navicular bone).

   a. He had no pain there either as I pressed.

In fact, his ankle was hardly swollen. He walked with only a slight limp. Adding up his score using the Ottawa ankle rules, he would not require an x-ray. In my own mind, I further questioned why he needed a referral to a subspecialty sports medicine clinic for this minor injury. I felt competent in treating this minor injury and involving physical therapy if required.

"I still want an x-ray and a referral to sports medicine for his injury," his father demanded. I had to hold my tongue from saying, Let's call an emergency helicopter for immediate transport.

The x-ray was negative for a fracture, and I made the referral after placing his ankle in a splint. I discussed the use of ice and elevation to reduce any swelling that might develop. Now I had to fill out a set of forms for the referral to sports medicine clinic. It felt awkward dictating a referral letter for this injury; but I did it, thinking, the cost of this care is more than necessary.

In this case, I acted as a triage officer by filling out forms, dictating a letter, and sending this patient to the sports medicine clinic.

This father felt high-tech care for his son's sprained ankle was essential because, in his eyes, his son may be looking at a college scholarship and perhaps even an NBA contract someday. He expected high-tech care would prevent disability and loss of these opportunities. I understood this. However, I did not think the outcome would be that much different comparing primary care to specialty clinic care for this minor injury.

I also knew of a few other facts pitting reality against cost in this case. This patient was only a high school sophomore. During the 2015–2016 high school athletic season, overall, a little over seven percent of high school athletes (about one in fourteen) go on to play a varsity sport in college. Approximately two percent of high school athletes (one in fifty) go on to play at the NCAA Division I level. Of course, these statistics are for all sports; and for basketball alone, the chance of playing NCAA Division I is 0.9%. The chances of a high school basketball player making it to the NBA are about three in ten thousand or 0.03%.

I had other athletic requests throughout the year that were like this father's demand. It seemed silly to me to be sending all these patients for expensive specialty care for minor injuries. But that was the expectation with these patients, or at least for their parents.

The urban standard of care encouraged these types of referrals from primary care to specialty care, which also included the transfer of responsibility for such things as diabetes (to endocrinology), asthma (to an allergist), emphysema (to the lung specialist), and the like. These specialists were much more accessible to the patients.

In my previous medical practice, I did not hesitate to transfer challenging cases to a specialist. I respected the knowledge of my colleagues in specialized areas when a diagnosis was in question, when there was no response to treatment, when the disease was complex, rare, or severe, or when a specialized skill was necessary. I knew my limitations and never got into trouble. However, I previously took care of many patients with diabetes, asthma, emphysema, and sprained ankles and most of the time, they did just fine. If I was not getting the result we desired, I referred. I was never litigated, and my patient satisfaction levels were always reported as being high.

This urban type of care system where referral is encouraged and expected raises the price of healthcare. Family physicians, general internists, and general pediatricians can manage many of these patients independently, and at less cost, when a case is routine and uncomplicated.

Not to suggest that all urban patients request referrals, but I noted these requests in a higher proportion than in rural folks. Many specialty physicians, business executives, patients, and medical students in training consequently saw primary care as more of an "urban triage officer" who is there to refer—quite a different perception of a primary care physician than what I had experienced in a small-town environment.

In small-town practice, most of the time folks resisted referral to specialty practices and very much respected and trusted their primary care physician. Rural patients sometimes tried to press me to do things I felt *should* merit referral to a specialty practice.

It is no wonder the "triage officer" perception of primary care was the myth generated in urban medical schools and specialty-oriented hospitals and clinics. It is what everyone saw as the job of a family physician, general internist, or general pediatrician from day to day. Respect for primary care seemed lower in urban culture. This sense encouraged medical students to choose a specialty with more honor and respect, and compensated better financially, than the primary care physician.

As I became acclimated to my new environment, I enjoyed the people I worked with; but the patient care system would take some getting used to.

Chapter 16

An Academic Project

ONE MUST ATTEND TO FOUR AREAS IN A PHYSI-
cian academic faculty job: patient care, teaching,
administration, and research. I felt adept at patient
care. My rural practice experience led to good teaching
reviews by the residents and interns. I knew nothing
about, nor had training in, research, public speaking,
curriculum development, and academic administration.

Enter Dr. John Beasley, an experienced faculty physician based at my residency clinic. John had a knack for
helping new faculty develop into their role as a teacher.
John approached me to find out how I was doing in my
new job.

My background in emergency cases in pediatrics,
medicine, and OB/GYN in rural practice resulted in
my certification in many life support courses: neonatal
resuscitation, pediatric advanced life support, advanced
trauma life support, and advanced cardiac life support.
I taught advanced cardiac life support and loved it.

One afternoon, Dr. Beasley and I went to lunch after
morning clinic.

"You know, John, I really appreciate you helping me
acclimate to my new job," I said. "Here's an idea I have.

See what you think. With all the life support courses out there, it is surprising that maternity care was left out. It is a common fact that obstetricians locate in urban areas and teaching centers near neonatal intensive care units. They do not locate in small towns. I practiced ten years in Reedsburg without an obstetrician on our hospital staff. Low-risk obstetric care in small communities is the primary responsibility of family physicians and nurse midwives."

"Jim, I agree," John responded. "Our challenge in the future is to fire-up family physicians and nurse midwives to offer maternity care; not only in these smaller communities but nationwide."

My enthusiasm increased. "Family physicians appear to be dropping OB nationwide. I'm sure there are many reasons for this," I said. "Lack of role models in residency, lifestyle issues, office disruption during the daytime, and perhaps fear of emergencies. Family physicians who practice in smaller communities often don't have an obstetrician to back them up when an obstetric emergency happens with a low-risk delivery. Take, for example, postpartum hemorrhage, or when the baby shoulders get stuck like a case I once had."

John's eyes widened, the volume of his voice increased, and he sat up. "Jim, I think this is an area we might focus on."

I went home that night and wrote about many of the emergency obstetric cases I had encountered in rural practice. I wrote down the use of forceps and vacuum instrument deliveries, delivering breech babies and other malpresentations and malpositions, stuck baby shoulders (shoulder dystocia), postpartum hemorrhage, and, yes, the one case I had with vasa previa and fetal death. In my mind, I could attach a name and face to each chapter of a possible syllabus.

I developed an outline of a two-day course using Advanced Cardiac Life Support (ACLS) and Advanced Trauma Life Support (ATLS) as templates. ACLS and ATLS both have a lecture section in the morning followed by afternoon practical workstations, using manikins. At the end of the two days, a written and practical test with certification followed.

What would we call such a maternity course? We wondered. Life support courses for infants, children, and adults already existed. *How about calling it the ALSO course (**Advanced Life Support in Obstetrics**)?*

Dr. John Beasley and I put on a few pounds going out for lunch together over the next several months as we tweaked my outline together.

"Jim, one thing you might do is present this outline at the Society of Teachers of Family Medicine (STFM) Annual National Convention," John suggested. "There is a family-centered perinatal subgroup within STFM. It would be good for your academic portfolio and faculty development."

I had no idea what STFM was, but John helped me get registered as a speaker.

People in the department helped me develop slides for my talk. This was before PowerPoint presentations.

The day of my presentation finally arrived. Nervous, I walked into the room. Fifty to sixty doctors I didn't know stood around talking to each other. One of them must have sensed my discomfort. Dr. Steve Ratcliffe kindly introduced himself and made me feel comfortable.

Finally, there was a call to order, and the officiator introduced me to the group by saying, "As everyone knows, rural communities have a maternity care access crisis looming. Obstetricians rarely locate in small towns. They are trained to deal with higher risk cases and prefer to be near neonatal intensive care units located in urban areas where delivery volume is also higher. Our first presentation today comes from the University of Wisconsin Department of Family Medicine. Dr. James Damos will present an idea for an obstetric course that focuses on treatment of emergencies that can result even with low-risk deliveries."

The audience clapped as I walked up to the microphone. I began clicking the remote for the slide machine. I don't remember much else. I was convinced the audience could tell I was a real amateur. Many of these doctors were skilled teachers of medicine. They could probably tell this was on-the-job training on how to present a topic.

Afterward, the faculty mobbed me. Many of the physician faculty said they would love to contribute as authors to the chapters I proposed for the course. They thought this was a great idea. Perhaps by standardizing a maternity care curriculum, the fear factor involving childbirth emergencies might be alleviated.

I returned home with many names for chapter authors in the new ALSO provider course. We began communicating over a new thing called computer email, and the ALSO provider course was born.

Chapter 17

ALSO Course Is a Movement

LINDA HAS SAID THAT I WORKED ON THE Advanced Life Support in Obstetrics (ALSO) course during the preparing of meals for the family. She felt cooking aromas inspired creative thoughts. The one computer we owned was in our kitchen. As parents, we could monitor what our children were doing on it while we performed kitchen chores.

I often came home after work with communication from those who had volunteered to write chapters in our proposed syllabus. I was the first (and second) editor of this course and worked with each author on their sections. My time on the computer was before supper in the evening. Over the next year, the ALSO course matured, and we had our first completed syllabus.

We presented our first two-day Advanced Life Support in Obstetrics (ALSO) course in 1991 at the Edgewater Hotel in Madison, Wisconsin. Many of the physicians who had written chapters in the syllabus came to lecture on their material and teach afternoon workstations. Dr. Beasley invited staff from the American Academy of Family Physicians to attend the course. The course was a big hit.

Later, Dr. Beasley and I traveled to Woodstock, New York, to work with the Simulaids Company to develop manikins for the course. We needed these marionettes for teaching instrument deliveries and other maneuvers required during difficult childbirth presentations. The engineers from Simulaids were excellent to work with.

Shortly after that first course in Madison at the Edgewater Hotel, our group of teachers/authors began getting invites to travel around the United States to present the ALSO educational skills in different areas of the country. The American Academy of Family Physicians assisted us in many ways with advertising, booking flights, meals, and hotel accommodations.

After extensive travel to teach the course, our original teaching group was getting tired. We had traveled to the East Coast, West Coast, around the Midwest, the South, and even to Alaska. All the travel was taking its toll.

We considered what we could do to keep this success going. These were the "barnstorming days." The success of this campaign indicated to us that there was a societal need. We developed a rather long-running list of medical centers requesting our teaching services. Like the other life support courses, we designed an ALSO instructor course to train more teachers. The ALSO movement was expanding.

In 1993, while all this occurred, Dr. Beasley, Dr. Rich Roberts (a physician and lawyer on the faculty in our department), and I met with staff from the American Academy of Family Physicians (AAFP) at O'Hare Airport to discuss their purchasing of the course. The AAFP later bought the course and developed an "ALSO Division" in their offices in Kansas City. A "board of directors" formed and physician board members updated the course regularly. Term limits with these board physicians injected a diversity of opinions into the curriculum. The administrative staff developed a budget, worked on improving manikins and the syllabus, and created a calendar of courses around the United States.

The AAFP ALSO division and the physicians and nurses who worked improving the course did an excellent job. The ALSO course, at the time of this writing, has now trained more than 70,000 maternity care providers in the U.S. alone since 1993, and more than 160,000 worldwide have completed training in over sixty countries. Over 3000 instructors have been trained. The ALSO course is now becoming a standard part of most family medicine residency curriculums. This may help rural access to maternity care. The course is teaching nurses, obstetric residents, and other emergency personnel around the world. Like the way the airline industry shows pilots how to handle emergencies in simulators, the ALSO course teaches obstetrical providers how to manage crises that can take place in the maternal delivery room (or in the ambulance on the way to the hospital).

The ALSO course won awards in London and in Canada, and later an international ALSO group developed. One obstetrician (Dr. Kim Hinshaw) from London wrote a letter recommending the ALSO course for the Bill and Melinda Gates award for Global Health.

Dr. Beasley and I served for five years on the first ALSO board of directors at the American Academy of Family Physicians. Later, we helped with the formation of the first ALSO international board involving obstetricians, nurse midwives, and family physicians from the U.S., Great Britain, and Canada.

The international committee has since expanded as the American Academy of Family Physicians has taken the course to new heights, including the development of a BLSO course (Basic Life Support in Obstetrics). Dr. Lee Dresang and Dr. Ann Evensen from the University of Wisconsin Department of Family Medicine became involved with the ALSO course. They and Dr. Larry Leeman from the University of New Mexico, and many others who have served on the board of directors have been instrumental in the further development of the ALSO model. A nurse by the name of Diana Winslow deserves an enormous amount of praise for the work she did directing the ALSO division at the AAFP. They and the board members did an excellent job refining and updating the syllabus and format.

This project has been a successful, collaborative movement initiated by family physicians and the American Academy of Family Physicians (AAFP). It took some time to get the American College of Obstetrics and Gynecology (ACOG) to recognize the course. Although many individual obstetricians participated in teaching the ALSO course, there was one who really stood out as someone who recognized the problem of maternity care shortages in underserved areas.

Dr. Steve Eisinger, an obstetrician/gynecologist, also managed a family medicine obstetric fellowship at the University of Rochester that trained family medicine residents beyond their three-year residency, including teaching the skill of cesarean section. Dr. Eisinger sat on our initial ALSO advisory board and served as a link between OB/GYN and Family Medicine as well as providing help with curriculum development. I have the utmost respect for this man. Dr. Steve became a good friend, whom I not only enjoyed working with but also hiking in the mountains with when we taught together out West.

One weekend, we invited the president of the American College of Obstetrics and Gynecology (ACOG) to one of our ALSO board meetings. We met every four to six months in different locations in the United States. We hoped we could collaborate and bring all providers of maternity care together (obstetricians, family physicians, nurse midwives, obstetric nurses, etc.). ACOG had not been very supportive of the course up until then. They did not fully support family physicians providing maternity care.

The president of ACOG sat at our meeting and was silent as we discussed maternity topics in the syllabus throughout the afternoon. When we got to the section of the curriculum on the use of forceps and vacuum instruments to assist delivery of the baby, he began to shift uncomfortably in his seat.

He finally interrupted one of the family physicians and said emphatically in a loud voice, "Family physicians should not do instrument deliveries. This chapter should be eliminated from the syllabus."

Of course, we all went silent and looked at each other.

I broke the silence. "When I was in Reedsburg, Wisconsin, we had no obstetrician on staff at our hospital for the ten years I was there. For most of our women, Reedsburg was an hour or more travel from Madison. What should I have done when a mother was exhausted from pushing or had progressive non-reassuring fetal heart tones and needed an instrument delivery to help mom deliver the baby? I had many of these situations in my rural practice. The alternative was a cesarean section on someone when it might be unnecessary.

"I guess we could close the obstetric unit at our rural hospital and request everyone drive an hour and a half to Madison for prenatal care and delivery. Long distance travel would not be ideal for these women. Recruitment of a functional obstetric group to our smaller community hospital seemed impossible. Many rural communities do not have enough deliveries to support the number of obstetricians needed to create an acceptable lifestyle.

"Also, these rural hospitals don't have neonatal intensive care units and on-staff neonatologists to deal with sicker babies. Obstetricians are used to dealing with higher risk cases in their training. It is nice to have a neonatologist available when these babies are born. Many obstetricians feel over-trained for these rural communities. As a family physician, I did not try to be a hero and handle high-risk cases in my small-town setting. I referred these cases to larger medical centers."

Despite my comments, he kept looking down and repeating loudly, "Family physicians should not do instrument deliveries." He continued to inform us that family physicians should not manage some of the other obstetric conditions outlined in the syllabus.

We moved on during the meeting, realizing he had sent us a signal that we would get no help from the American College of Obstetrics and Gynecology.

Years later, a University of Wisconsin–Baraboo rural family medicine resident physician and I published an article in the journal, *American Family Physician,* entitled "Vacuum-assisted Vaginal Delivery" (Christina D. Hook, James R. Damos, *American Family Physician* 78(8):953–60, October 2008). How to do an instrument delivery using a vacuum unit is the topic of this journal commentary.

An obstetrician in London emailed me saying this article is now one model for teaching vacuum deliveries to obstetricians in the United Kingdom, along with the ALSO workshop on instrument deliveries that I co-authored for the Advanced Life Support in Obstetrics (ALSO) syllabus.

So much for "Family physicians should not do instrument deliveries."

When the ALSO course became international and started winning awards in other countries, a new president from the American College of Obstetrics and Gynecology became more involved with the American Academy of Family Physicians. It was great to see ACOG now engaged with the ALSO movement. Collaboration, not competition, has always been the goal. Getting ACOG and the AAFP working together with the nursing profession in a collaborative way improves rural maternity access to healthcare.

The University of Wisconsin Obstetrics and Gynecology Department has now developed a rural OB/GYN training track with a focus on training OB/GYN physicians for rural Wisconsin. This is one of the first in the nation, and it is fantastic to see. I believe OB/GYN physicians and family physicians can work together in smaller communities and offer excellent care.

In contrast to what is seen in the United States, family physicians, obstetricians, and nurse midwives from the United Kingdom have always been collaborative and extremely helpful with the development of the ALSO course. They helped spur the growth of ALSO International, along with physicians and nurses from Canada. The film *Save Mom—ALSO in Africa* was awarded the London Independent Film Award in 2017.

To end this chapter, yes, I believe family medicine does contribute to medical education. Another myth busted.

Chapter 18

Starting to Crave Rural Practice Again

THE ALSO COURSE DEVELOPMENT AND SUBSE-
quent ALSO teaching were an incredibly gratifying eight-year period for me in academics. Linda and
I had an opportunity to travel throughout the United
States and meet many interesting people from Canada,
the United Kingdom, Mexico, and some of the South
American countries.

Jenny was now in college at the University of
Wisconsin–Madison. She loved children, received training and became a therapist for children with autism as
a job while in school. She was interested in becoming a
school psychologist. Tim was ready to leave for college
soon. He aspired to become a journalist.

In my academic job, I enjoyed teaching and working
with the many talented people from the University of
Wisconsin Department of Family Medicine. In 1991, the
faculty voted me in as the Madison residency program
director, and I served in this position for three years all
while editing, writing, and traveling with the developing ALSO course, continuing to teach, and seeing my

own patient panel at the clinic. These were busy but rewarding times.

Unfortunately, I had difficulty adapting to the urban patient care system and urban culture that I found so different from my previous practice. It just wasn't my cup of tea. It appeared more chaotic, specialty-oriented, lacking in continuity of patient care, and expensive. I missed small-town medical practice and its autonomy, family approaches, and patient continuity. To me, maternity care, labor, and delivery were more rewarding in the smaller community hospital.

An example of an urban family physician-obstetrician interaction occurred on one Sunday evening. A resident and I followed a patient in labor most of the day at one of the larger private hospitals. Our patient progressed to having a fully dilated cervix. She began pushing but was having trouble bringing the baby's head down. After two hours of pushing, it was the urban standard of care that we obtain a consultation with an obstetrician.

We already had this young lady pushing in different positions; we emptied her bladder, and we carefully monitored the baby for signs of non-reassuring heart tones through electronic fetal monitoring. We assessed her contraction pattern and added some Pitocin, a hormone that stimulates labor contractions. The baby did not appear unusually large, and I felt the mother's pelvis was adequate for vaginal delivery.

"I think we are supposed to consult an obstetrician, since it has been two hours of pushing," I said to the resident physician.

"I will check to see which obstetrician is in the hospital and taking consults," the resident replied. About ten minutes later, our consultation arrived. He was not very cordial.

"What is going on here?" he grumbled to the nurse while walking right by us. He examined our patient.

"I feel this baby is occiput posterior," the obstetrician groused. This is when the baby is looking up at the ceiling during delivery instead of coming out looking at the floor. We call this delivering "sunny side up," with the back of the baby's head against mom's tailbone.

Babies usually are delivered looking down at the floor. Occiput posterior babies have a more substantial part of the head (the occiput or back of the head) presenting. The head is not tucked in a flexed position looking down. Occiput posterior (looking up) babies have more difficulties delivering vaginally.

"We need to perform a forceps rotation to turn the baby," he said in a louder voice. He prepared to place forceps on the head and turn it around.

"Are you sure the baby is occiput posterior?" I questioned. "Mom has not been complaining of back pain, and I thought by my exam she was left occiput anterior (face looking down); a normal position. I think I can also feel the back of the baby's head just above mom's pubic bone on my abdominal exam."

He overruled me, grumbling, "This is a procedure I need to do. Family physicians should avoid it." He asked the nurse to set things up for the forceps rotation in a delivery room separate from the labor area.

Once we got back to the delivery area, he used specialized forceps called Keiland forceps to turn the baby's head. It turned out to be a challenging delivery. He had difficulty rotating the head and finally pulled the baby out occiput posterior (looking up at the ceiling). He had turned the baby from a normal to an abnormal position. His hands shook as he pulled on the head. This resulted in a post-partum hemorrhage from a vaginal laceration, which he repaired. The mother sustained an injury that tore into her rectum (a fourth-degree tear), which he had to fix. The baby underwent resuscitation by the on-call neonatologist who the obstetrician summoned. The baby recovered. The obstetrician did not say much. The room was silent as he sutured the vaginal lacerations and repaired the patient's rectum.

When he finished, he passed by me, glared and whispered in my ear, "That sometimes happens. Cool it."

In rural practice, I had no obstetrician on staff with me. I would have spoken with this young lady about her stamina and let her continue to push if the baby was doing well and she continued to make some progress, even though it was two hours. We would have monitored the baby for signs of distress.

After trying squat pushing, different maternal positions, and making sure the bladder was empty, I may have, with her consent, placed a vacuum unit on the baby's head and delivered the baby that way.

The vacuum unit does not have "blades" inside the woman's vagina, and it will pop off if there is a tight squeeze that could cause injury. We were just becoming familiar with the use of the vacuum unit at the end of my time in Reedsburg. I would not attempt a forceps rotation since I was not trained in that skill.

Another rural option would be a cesarean section if the mother became exhausted and/or there were non-reassuring fetal heart tones. I sensed my rural choices would have led to less morbidity for this mom.

This experience was an unusual encounter. Most of the obstetricians I worked with were collegial and helpful. However, this case got me thinking about a move back to rural medical practice.

I read that a Society of Teachers of Family Medicine study on rural health showed that the longer a resident physician trained in a small community learning medicine, the higher the placement in subsequent small-town practice.

Months spent in a rural area for training	Percent of Graduates in the program choosing rural practice
0	24%
1	37%
2	46%
3	52%
6	51%
+22	69%

From "Family practice residency programs and the graduation of rural family physicians" by Bowman RC, Penrod JD.

I started thinking about creating a physician rural training program. By doing so, I could move back to small-town practice, the culture I preferred while continuing to teach.

After inquiring with several communities (including my old Reedsburg community) and meeting with several hospital administrations and medical staffs, the rural practice in Baraboo, Wisconsin, was the most enthusiastic about having a residency training program based in their town. The administration and physician staff in Baraboo appeared eager to enter a relationship with the University of Wisconsin Department of Family Medicine. Baraboo (population around 12,000) was about one hour north of Madison.

We assembled a team to work on establishing a rural physician training program. As the curriculum came to fruition, Linda and I considered moving to Baraboo, Wisconsin.

Teaching and Practicing Rural Medicine

Chapter 19

The Move

ENTER DR. BOB AND GINNY KOTTKAMP AGAIN, the friends from our St. Louis medical school days who visited us when we contemplated moving from Reedsburg to Madison. Bob and Ginny had just moved to Ludlow, Vermont, and enjoyed living in a smaller community. They provided support as we contemplated this new move.

Once again, Linda and I drew a line down the middle of a piece of paper. We considered the pros and cons, and the move to Baraboo won out. We destroyed the alternatives.

We moved, and I began working at the clinic in Baraboo. My job consisted of seeing patients, teaching resident physicians in training, and serving as program director of the University of Wisconsin–Baraboo physician rural training program. I taught utilizing the expanded set of medical practice skills I had developed in my residency, and in Reedsburg for ten years.

It was a Saturday, and I was on-call for the Baraboo Clinic during a graduation picnic for the first graduates of the Baraboo Rural Training Track. I agreed to take

the call so the rest of the Baraboo faculty could participate in the graduation ceremonies. I was told Saturdays
could be busy, but I would likely be able to attend the
picnic. Those were famous last words.

I had six hospital admissions that afternoon. A tourist visiting the area from Chicago came in, in active
labor although two weeks from her due date. She had
ruptured her membranes at one of the water parks in
the Wisconsin Dells. She went on to a spontaneous vaginal delivery without complication.

Other admissions were more complicated. I admitted a gentleman in congestive heart failure; an elderly
woman with a hip fracture from a fall who needed to be
evaluated medically before surgery by our orthopedist;
someone with diarrhea and dehydration; and a middle-
aged man admitted for a chest pain evaluation, who did
not have convincing evidence of a heart attack.

The most difficult challenge was a twenty-three-
year-old male who came in with a fever of 102°, a cough,
and difficulty breathing.

The ER doctor called, "Jim, I have a very sick young
man here." When I arrived at the hospital emergency
room, I reviewed his chest x-ray. It was quite impressive.
He had bilateral (both lungs) pneumonia with what
looked like abscesses (like boils) in each lung.

We started an IV, placed him on oxygen, did blood,
urine, and sputum cultures, and started him on broad-
spectrum antibiotics, including coverage for staph and
gram-negative pneumonia. He did not look good. Due
to his young age and deteriorating condition, I made

the decision to transfer him to Madison. His medical insurance dictated that he be transported to the University Hospital, and transfer via helicopter was arranged. The old traveling intensive care unit buses were now extinct.

I later heard the patient's status declined to the point of being on a respirator, and it was discovered he was HIV positive. He was hospitalized for several weeks but survived. The University Hospital was good at keeping me informed as to how he was doing. I was interested in how they worked up this young man and treated him. I used any information my consultants provided me, either by phone or by consult letter, to learn and fine-tune my own approaches to patient care.

That night, things finally calmed down by nine o'clock. Although I never made it to the picnic, it felt good to be back doing the things I loved in high volume.

I looked forward to sharing my knowledge and skills with interns/residents in the rural setting. I felt the smaller community learning laboratory was ready to be tapped for teaching medicine, and I could better maintain my hospital skills with a higher volume of cases all year long.

Chapter 20

Can You Stop by the Nursing Home Later?

ONE OF THE UNIQUE THINGS ABOUT PRIMARY care is that we have the opportunity and privilege of seeing people and problems of all kinds. This leads to a variety of experiences.

I had one patient named Helen who always asked about my fishing trips to Canada. She was in her nineties and dying, unfortunately, of aggressive cancer. In the nursing home and on hospice/palliative care, she remained remarkably upbeat and loved to talk fishing whenever I visited her. She and her husband had gone on many Canadian fishing trips over their sixty plus years of marriage.

One afternoon, I got a call from the nursing home. "Doctor, any chance you could stop by on your way home tonight? Helen really wants to talk to you. I'm not sure if the end is near or whether she's having some symptoms. She won't give me much information."

Helen was frail and had been in bed all day. The nursing home was one block from our clinic and easy to get to on my way home. No parking garages or traffic.

I got done with my last patient, finished my charting, then drove to the nursing home. When I arrived, the nurse accompanied me to the bedside. "Doctor, I'm not sure what's going on with her," the nurse said. "She has been requesting your attendance all day. I asked her if she's having pain, nausea, or any other symptoms and she has denied them. She will not tell me why she needs you."

As we entered the room, Helen sat up in bed with a big smile on her face. She looked ready to jump out of bed and do a victory dance, but I knew she was too weak to do so. She got the giggles and said, "Hello, Dr. Damos. If you will, could you grab that book under the chair over there?"

I grabbed the book and gave it to her.

"Now, come on, let's see what's inside. Sit down here next to me on the bed," Helen said with a beaming smile. The nurse looked on curiously, no doubt wondering what was inside the book.

Helen proudly showed me an old photo album her daughter had found at home. She told me to open the book. I did and set eyes on about twenty pages of Canadian fishing pictures.

I sat there for thirty minutes as Helen went through each page with me. She told the story behind the fish caught that day, and where in Canada that she and her husband had caught them.

She had a wonderful time reminiscing with me sitting at her bedside. Three days later, Helen died peacefully at the age of ninety-five.

Perhaps showing me her Canadian pictures was on a "bucket list" for her. This term evolved from the 2007 movie *The Bucket List* starring Jack Nicholson and Morgan Freeman. I observed over my career that patients with terminal illness often developed such bucket lists. As their life came to an end, completing a bucket list item seemed to bring closure for them, like the last chapter of a book.

Like the bass fisherman I treated who had pancreatic cancer, refused treatment, made amends with his brother and went on two vacations before he died, goal-setting in Helen's terminal illness brought her peace. As her long-time primary care physician, I felt privileged to help her accomplish this goal.

Chapter 21

Listen to the Patient, Confirm What You Hear and See

RETURNED TO WORK FROM A ONE-WEEK FAMILY vacation to a stressful first day back. Numerous lab results and x-ray reports waited on me, as well as calls from individuals who had questions that "only their own doctor could answer so have him call me when he gets back."

At eight a.m., I started the day making rounds in the hospital with one of our resident physicians in training, Dr. Bridget, a very bright, hardworking doctor who loves to learn.

Dr. Bridget and I noted we had one admission in the hospital scheduled for discharge. Our patient, a charming young lady who has been a long-term patient of mine, was admitted with vague weakness and tingling in her leg. A workup in the hospital included a history, physical exam, lab studies, x-rays, and an MRI of her lower spine. We note the workup was all negative, and she awaited discharge with a diagnosis of work-related anxiety and stress.

The paperwork and discharge instructions had already been filled out by the physician who followed her in my absence. She was ready to go.

I was familiar with our patient's history, which included several life-threatening health problems in the past. She always followed medical instructions religiously and was very health-minded. When she presented with symptoms, my red flags went up. This doctor-patient continuity should never be underestimated.

Dr. Bridget and I reviewed her workup in the chart and then went to see her. We wanted to do our own evaluation of her symptoms before discharging her.

"Bridget, why don't you take the history and do a neurological exam at the bedside, and I will observe you," I said.

As expected, Dr. Bridget did a competent history and physical exam, asking all the right questions. Our patient had neurologic symptoms of weakness in her left leg as well as decreased sensation to a pinprick. We noted her gait was affected when we had her walk. Dr. Bridget mapped out a dermatome, or a lumbar spine level, where she thought there might be an abnormality. I agreed.

"Let's go down to radiology and review her MRI," I said.

The MRI had been read as negative. Dr. Bridget and I noted that her physical findings indicated a spinal level higher than what the MRI had imaged. We expressed our concerns to the radiologist. We did not feel comfortable sending this patient home for outpatient follow-up. We were concerned she might fall with her unsteady gait. More importantly, we did not feel the MRI had looked at the area we worried about based on our exam.

We decided to order a repeat MRI of her spine to include a level a bit higher than what her previous MRI had imaged. The radiologist was very accommodating in getting our patient worked in that morning. We canceled her discharge pending the repeat MRI. Something did not appear right in matching the MRI findings with our own historical and physical results.

Dr. Bridget and I then went on to the clinic to see patients. A few hours later, my nurse Sue called me out of an exam room to answer a phone call from the hospital radiologist.

As I put the telephone to my ear and said hello, the radiologist said, "Jim, you and your resident physician are geniuses. You were obviously very thorough in your evaluation of her. She has a rather large spinal cord tumor noted at a higher level on the repeat MRI that did not show on the previous exam."

I called to let Bridget know what the findings were, and we returned to the hospital at lunchtime to inform our patient of the bad news.

Dr. Bridget did the talking. "I am afraid we have some bad news for you (warning shot fired—patient perks up). Your repeat MRI shows a spinal cord mass at a level higher than what the previous MRI had imaged. I wish I had better news for you. We would like to make a referral to a neurosurgeon in Madison and get going on this. Do you have any names in mind of a neuro-surgeon you trust, or would you want us to choose a neurosurgeon for you?"

"I will go with who you recommend. I trust your judgment," the patient replied.

We made a referral to a neurosurgeon, and she left for Madison for neurosurgery consultation. They took her right to the operating room, where she had a mass removed from her spinal cord.

She was told that even though this was a benign mass and not malignant, had she waited longer before attending to this, she may have ended up paralyzed for life and possibly in a wheelchair. The mass might have choked off blood supply to the spinal cord in that area.

She went through several months of physical ther-apy, walking initially with a walker, moving up to a cane, and finally walking naturally again.

The moral of this story is that a physician must do their own assessment and be thorough with taking the patient history and physical examination. The problem with this case was that the first MRI had missed the mass higher up in the spinal cord. We discovered this by trying to match her history and physical findings with the MRI that had been done. When they did not match, we questioned this disparity. I also suspected something else was going on (beyond stress/anxiety) knowing this patient's past and having been through some of these experiences with her. Having a long-term doctor-patient relationship is an advantage.

I remember one of my instructors saying to me in the past: "Listen to the patient, as they will tell you the diagnosis if you ask the right questions and you know them well. Your physical exam, labs, and imaging, then, will just confirm what you already know. Spend time with them. Learn."

Chapter 22

A Reminder Why I Became a Physician

I MADE HOUSE CALLS DURING MY ENTIRE THIRTY-six-year career. Some feel house calls are outdated and poorly compensated financially. They are a sign of the old "GP doctor" who many believe is a thing of the past. I disagree. There is much to be gained *for the patient* by making a house call. When I saw salt on the table, and bacon and ham in the refrigerator, I had a better perspective on why my patient with congestive heart failure was decompensating. When I was puzzled why my elderly patient with emphysema was having increasing difficulties breathing, a house call revealed a thermostat turned up to eighty degrees with no windows open. An office visit would have led to a nebulizer treatment, adjustment and patient education on the use of the patient's inhaler and perhaps a round of steroids prescribed, instead of opening some windows during a spring day and turning the heat down.

House calls offered comfort to a dying patient and saved the family the time of bringing a frail patient into the office. I felt a house call always led to a closer doctor-patient relationship, and I too benefited from my own feeling of having comforted someone through a house call.

❧

One of my favorite times of the year is Christmas, a spiritual season accompanied by family, friends, and charity. I envision warm fires, good food and drink, candlelight services, prayer, decorations, and excited, happy children.

Aside from the time I treated the child with bacterial tracheitis, another Christmas stands out for me. I saw my last patient in the office one evening a few days before Christmas Eve. After finishing my records, I was getting ready to go home when a call came in from a patient.

"Dr. Damos, I am afraid my wife is not doing well. As you know, she is dying of cancer and is in hospice, having exhausted all forms of treatment. And she is only forty-nine." His voice quivered over the phone as he spoke with me. I could tell he was scared. He continued, "I called the hospice nurse on call, but she is currently busy with another patient. My wife is unconscious, very restless, and I wonder if she is in pain. I have given her morphine dose to her, but it is not helping. I'm not sure if I should give more or not."

"I know where you live. I will stop by your house on my way home. I will be there within the half-hour," I said.

I flashed back to the nun who had sat with me during my daughter's cancer operation. She had been so empathic and comforting. I wanted to do the same for this man. I knew the feelings he must be experiencing.

I left the clinic and encountered a beautiful snow-fall: no wind and large snowflakes falling straight down. The epitome of the Christmas season—very spiritual, although visibility was almost nil.

I arrived at his home, where he met me, grief-stricken, at the front door. On the one hand, the Christmas season permeated the air with a beautiful snowfall happening on a still, cloudless night with the stars shining. On the other hand, a man is losing his companion, friend, and wife of many years at a time when there should be joy in the air.

As I entered his home, I saw his wife on the couch. She laid there in a fetal position, looking emaciated and near death. She was unconscious and moaning, unable to communicate.

I examined her, taking her blood pressure, pulse, and temperature. She had low blood pressure, a rapid and weak pulse, and fever. Dehydrated, she likely had pneumonia. Her distended abdomen was filled with fluid from her cancer; something we call "malignant ascites."

Her advanced directive indicated her preference to be kept comfortable without hospitalization. We reviewed this advanced directive, and her husband agreed. His primary concern was that she might be experiencing pain, but he did not know how much morphine he could give her without doing her harm.

Would it be euthanasia to give this patient more morphine to allay what her husband and I perceived as pain while she lay moaning on the couch? Too much morphine can cause a patient to stop breathing. Would we be a "death squad" if she stopped breathing and died with the extra doses of morphine?

There is an ethical doctrine or principle called the *"doctrine of double effect."* What this doctrine or principle says is that it is permissible to risk harm such as the death of a human being as a side effect to promoting good (relief of pain in this case with morphine). We are taught as physicians that in cases like this, there is no "ceiling dose" of morphine if you intend to relieve pain and not intentionally give a lethal dose (which I did not).

I did just that. I gave an extra dose of morphine on top of the previous milligrams that her husband had already given her. There are formulas we physicians use to calculate an increased amount to relieve pain—so-called breakthrough doses. I figured her breakthrough dose using her usual daily basal morphine dose.

I placed oxygen on her and changed her position on the couch, thinking that might make her more comfortable. She did not appear to have a distended bladder on examination, and I did not see any bedsores.

Her husband and I then sat down at the kitchen table to talk for a while and for me to watch for any effect of my interventions. I knew I might need to give her more morphine if she continued to show extreme behaviors. He made us both a cup of tea.

Over the next thirty minutes, her husband related their life story through his watery eyes. I listened as he narrated the last chapter of their married lives.

Finally, he said, "Doctor, we have had a great marriage. I love her so much. It is just awful to see her like this. I am going to miss her a lot. I don't know how I will go on. But I can't tell you how much I appreciate you coming to my home tonight. Thank you."

I replied, "I too feel sad and will miss her. I noted during her clinic visits that she was so kind and fun to be around. What I cherished most about both of you as a couple was the strength you showed throughout her illness. I can't tell you enough what a superb job you have done in caring for her. I feel privileged to have been able to serve as your doctor. You have taught me the art of caregiving. You should never doubt the job you have done in caring for her."

I tried to offer support with my words but, in these circumstances, actions speak louder than words. My house call and ability to just sit and listen to him was more important than anything I could have said. He needed to talk and express his feelings.

We underestimate the fear people have when they experience the death of a loved one alone. We undervalue the power of just listening to a patient or caregiver.

His wife settled down and appeared to be sleeping peacefully. While I was still there, the hospice nurse called back to say she had completed her other duties and was on her way over. As I left, he hugged me and thanked me for the "house call that most doctors no longer make."

I walked back into the Christmas snowfall with a warm but sad feeling in my heart. Although house calls are not "cost-effective," I learned this evening of their tremendous value to the patient and myself.

His wife died the next morning. I later received a beautiful card in the mail from the husband thanking me for what I had done. He said he would never forget this experience. I never did either. There was no charge for the visit.

Chapter 23

Rural Maternity Care and Resource Overload

SOME SAY SMALLER HOSPITALS ARE NOT BUSY enough and should close. There was a day I endured that illustrates why I disagree with this belief.

Most rural obstetrics is routine and has acceptable outcomes. It is the ten percent that leads to challenges. I had a patient past her due date. We had monitored her pregnancy closely with fetal monitoring (called fetal nonstress testing) and ultrasounds. These tests showed us we needed to get her delivered, and she was admitted to the hospital for induction of labor that evening. We performed cervical ripening with a vaginal insert medication called cervidil. The next morning, we decided to begin her on Pitocin, a hormone to initiate labor contractions.

The beautiful thing about our small-town practice was that the hospital OB unit was only a couple minute walk from my workplace. In fact, her labor room window was just opposite my clinic office window on a second floor. The nurse could literally wave to me and hold up numbers for how far dilated the patient was.

My patient spent the day in labor, and after the clinic day wound down, I dropped by the OB unit to see how my patient was doing. She had progressed throughout the day to around six to seven centimeters dilated, and everything looked good.

I called home. "Linda, I'll eat here at the hospital. I have a lady in labor six to seven centimeters dilated who will likely deliver soon. Go ahead with dinner, and I'll see you later this evening." A familiar scenario to Linda; she wished me luck.

I had a dinner of hospital cafeteria food, chatted with some of the nursing staff for a while and went back upstairs to check on this soon-to-be mother.

She had progressed to completely dilated and felt like pushing.

Over the next hour, she felt a lot of back pain. The baby's head had not descended into the pelvis like I wanted it to. As I examined her, I thought the baby presented occiput posterior, the "sunny side up," position previously described as looking at the ceiling with the back of the baby's head against mom's tailbone.

The nurse tried shifting mom into different positions (to try and rotate the head naturally) while the mom pushed. She also used a "squat bar" which allows mom to squat in a sort of sitting position, holding onto a bar in front of her. This flattens the tailbone and makes for more room in the pelvis. I made sure mom's bladder was empty so that a large, full bladder didn't compete with the head for space in the pelvis. At one point, I tried to manually rotate the baby's head into a normal position, but this was unsuccessful.

As mom pushed, we noted that the baby's heart tones began to drop lower and lower with each push. These deteriorating fetal heart tones started to have more delayed recovery back to baseline after the contraction was over. These changes can be a sign that the baby feels the stress of labor.

I placed oxygen on the mom and tried changing her position. I turned off the Pitocin hormone drip to give baby and mom a break. I checked mom vaginally to see if anything else had changed. I notified my physician partner on call that I would need him to attend to the baby at birth. He was on standby.

Shortly after that, we noted mom's pulse increasing, and her blood pressure dropping. She began complaining of lower abdominal pain in between contractions. I gave her a fluid challenge, and ordered lab tests, concerned about a condition called placental abruption. Placental abruption is when the placenta (afterbirth) wholly or partially separates from the mom's uterus before the baby is born. This is quite serious and can decrease the amount of oxygen and nutrients to the baby. It can cause maternal bleeding. This was probably the cause of mom's fall in blood pressure, increased pulse, and the non-reassuring fetal heart tones.

After the fluid challenge to mom, and because the baby remained in the occiput posterior position with the head still a bit higher in the pelvis for an instrument delivery, I said to the nurse, "We need to arrange for an emergency cesarean section."

I informed mom of my thinking and what needed to be done. Things were deteriorating and not looking good. The nurse left to start calling people and get urgent help.

A few minutes later, the nurse returned to tell me she had terrible news. "They have just brought in multiple victims from a car accident. All the operating rooms, surgeons, and anesthetists are tied up. We are trying to contact another anesthetist from a nearby hospital to come in. Hopefully, an operating room will be available shortly."

We now had what I coined "rural hospital resource overload"—our staff and facility overloaded with critical patients.

I re-examined the patient to find the baby's head lower in the pelvis but still in the abnormal position of occiput posterior. I asked to put on the vacuum unit to try to do an instrument delivery. I would attach a suction cup to the baby's head and try to pull the baby out. Sometimes one will see a rotation of the baby's head to a normal anterior (face down) position as the doctor pulls with the vacuum. It is safer than forceps since there are no blades inside mom's vagina.

I had no trouble placing the vacuum unit on the baby; but as I pulled, the suction gave away, and the cup popped off. I reapplied the vacuum cup, making sure I applied it as far posterior as I could, only to have it pop off again as I pulled. I attempted this one more time. Our rule is "three strikes, and you're out."

I gently tugged while mom pushed. It popped off a third time.

Remembering three pop-offs may indicate the baby's head is prominent, leading to a tight squeeze coming through the pelvis, I was thinking more than ever that an emergency Cesarean section may be needed. It is recommended not to try forceps after a failed vacuum delivery.

I checked with the nurse. "Do we have an operating room yet?"

She replies, "Sorry, not yet. No operating room or anesthetist."

In the interim, nothing had changed. The baby's heart tones now were in the sixties and not improving.

My choices at this point were threefold. First, I could proceed with a cesarean section under local anesthesia at the bedside. Second, I could try to pull the baby out with forceps, even though it is frowned upon as potentially being dangerous and harmful after a failed vacuum extraction. Third, I can do nothing. I already had tried manual rotation of the head.

Doing nothing is unacceptable. In fact, all three choices are undesirable.

I felt comfortable with forceps, having done many forceps deliveries over the years. I had assisted with many cesarean sections but did not feel I had the experience to do one myself alone—especially under local anesthesia at the bedside. Our general surgeons did all the cesarean sections in our rural community. We had no obstetrician on staff.

I chose option number two. I placed Simpson forceps on the baby's head and began to artfully pull, using what we taught in the ALSO course. I had been a co-author of the chapter on instrument delivery. As

I applied the blades and began to pull, I found I could deliver the baby. I used a little different technique than the usual forceps procedure since the baby was occiput posterior. I pulled the baby out "sunny side up." The forceps operation worked; the baby delivered. At this point, nursing staff, an emergency room physician and my family physician partner had arrived. We all began to work on the baby, who was not breathing and entirely limp. We also were attending to mom at the same time.

The baby's pulse was around 60 (average should be approximately 120 for this baby), and we began CPR. The ER doc successfully intubated the baby's windpipe and started breathing for her. We put a catheter into the baby's umbilical vein and gave a fluid challenge of saline solution (10 ccs/kilogram). Finally, we provided the baby with a dose of epinephrine (adrenaline) into the umbilical vein. Her pulse picked up and rose to around 115. We continued to breathe for the baby with the Ambu bag.

I attended to mom and delivered her placenta. This was sent to pathology. It later showed an abruption of the placenta, just as we had suspected.

We called a regional neonatal intensive care unit to begin a transfer of the baby. They recommended "hypothermic therapy." Research has found that cooling a baby to around 91–92° temperature for three days after birth is a treatment for a condition called *"hypoxic-ischemic encephalopathy."* This cooling treatment reduces brain damage, improves survival, and hopefully reduces disability in the future.

By now, other people had arrived to help us out. One of the surgeons had completed what he was doing with the auto accident victims and came upstairs. A nurse anesthetist arrived in the obstetric unit to help. When contacted, our local pediatrician came in without hesitation despite being on vacation.

These people were not on call, yet they came in to assist. This is the culture of rural health, where doctors work together for the good of the patient even though they are not on call.

The neonatal team arrived within the next ninety minutes to transfer our baby. We had continued to breathe for the baby. In the meantime, we had done other studies, such as checking the baby's blood sugar, electrolytes, and blood count. We obtained a chest x-ray to check for a collapsed lung and to check for the endotracheal tube placement. We started an IV for IV fluids. Upon the phone advice of the neonatologist, we had cooled the baby to a rectal temperature of around 93° by the time they arrived.

I thanked my rural team for their help and returned home. I did not sleep well, but I needed to get up in two hours to see clinic patients despite the excitement from last night.

I did not feel right about this case. I had been backed into a corner with "rural hospital resource overload."

Mom was okay, but I felt apprehensive about the baby. I would feel awful if this baby ended up disabled in some way.

The next morning, I called the neonatal intensive care unit to see how the baby was doing. Often, the staffs at these larger centers do not understand the challenges we have in rural communities, and they can be quite rude with us doctors when we call to find out how our referrals are doing. Some small-town doctors don't phone because of the way they are treated.

However, when I phoned this NICU, several neonatal intensive care unit nurses *and* the neonatologist spoke to me in a supportive, collegial manner. The neonatologist told me the baby exhibited what might be some seizure activity. They were doing an imaging study on the baby's head to make sure there was no internal hemorrhage or injury from the forceps after attempting vacuum delivery unsuccessfully. My heart sank.

I later called again that afternoon and was relieved to find out that I had caused no internal head bleeding or visible damage from the forceps or vacuum delivery. A pediatric neurologist assessed the baby and felt this was not seizure activity but, instead, shivering from the hypothermic cooling therapy.

Several days later, the baby was feeding well, looked good, and was discharged after a total of five days hospitalized.

Fast forward several years later, when this beautiful little girl came into the office for a well-child visit. Sharp, cute, interactive, with an undeniable bond with her mom which is very strong.

We should not close rural hospitals. There is a need out here.

Chapter 24

Tough Mary

MARY LIVED ON A FARM AND WORKED RIGHT alongside her husband milking cows, caring for steers, harvesting crops, and providing for her family. Mary would come into our hospital in labor having had no prenatal care and often very close to delivering. I suspected her lack of prenatal care related to her lack of health insurance. She would usually pay cash for the delivery, and you would not see her again until her next childbirth. I delivered three of her children. The third time was the most memorable.

While seeing patients one afternoon in the clinic, I received a call from the hospital that Mary had arrived in labor and feeling "pushy." This urgent call meant Mary was ready to deliver. Again, I had not seen her for any prenatal care.

I told my clinic nurse, Sue (a great nurse to work with), what was happening so she could inform the patients and give them the option of waiting or rescheduling. Usually, with Mary, it would not be too long anyway.

As I arrived in labor and delivery, I saw Mary with her legs up and the nurse trying to coach her. But "Tough Mary" was not cooperating.

I quickly washed my hands, put on a gown and gloves, and tried to coach Mary with pushing.

As labor started, I said, "Come on, Mary, a contraction has started. The head is right there, and if you push, we will get this baby delivered."

With a scowl on her face, she replied emphatically, "NO! Every time I push, my tooth hurts."

As I looked in her mouth, I saw a severely decayed tooth, with the surrounding gum inflamed. She appeared to have dental caries and probably a dental abscess in one tooth. I tried to convince her that one push would deliver this baby.

Mary pounded her fists against her thighs and breathing deeply, emphatically stated, "I told you Doc, my tooth hurts!"

I asked the nurse if she could get a tube of lidocaine gel. Lidocaine is an anesthetic, and I thought if we applied this to the tooth area, perhaps it would deaden the pain just enough to allow Mary to push. The nurse left the room to see what she could find.

At this point, I saw Mary frown, grunt, and loudly growl. She reached into her mouth, grabbed the decayed tooth, and pulled as hard as she could while shaking her head from side to side. She pulled the tooth out and threw it across the room in disgust.

This event angered her husband standing by her side. He said, "Don't throw that away, you idiot!"

I'm not sure what he planned to do with it, but he quickly retrieved the extracted tooth off the floor and put it in his pocket. At that point, our patient gave one long, massive push, and the baby delivered with excellent Apgars of 9 and 10 (as usual for "Tough Mary"). The Apgar score rates the baby's Appearance (color), Pulse, Grimace (reflex irritability), Activity (muscle tone) and Respiratory rate, assigning 0–2 points to each item with a final score of 1–10. A score of 7–10 is normal and indicates the baby is doing well.

Of course, there was no episiotomy. Mary had no vaginal lacerations or visible childbirth injury. The placenta was delivered without complication after I administered some oxytocin and applied traction on the umbilical cord. Mary had no postpartum hemorrhage. All went well.

As usual, Mary requested to leave and go home at this point. We convinced her to stay to follow our group B streptococcus protocol. Group B streptococcus is a bacterium that may live in about twenty-five percent of healthy women's vaginas or rectums. Women who test positive with these bacteria can pass these bacteria on to their infant, potentially causing a severe infection. A hospital protocol is used to prevent this which may include administering antibiotics during labor. Mary had no prenatal care, no prenatal group B strep screening, and no time to administer antibiotics during labor.

She agreed to stay, finally, after some coaxing. After forty-eight hours of placing the baby on our protocol, she was packed and ready to go when I came for rounds. Number three was brought into the world. Mary would likely be milking cows tonight when she arrived home.

Ah yes, rural maternity care is always exciting.

Chapter 25

Haiti Medical Mission

I T WAS 2002. I CONTINUED TO ENJOY PRACTICING medicine, teaching and serving as the program director in our University of Wisconsin–Baraboo Physician Rural Training Program which had become one national model for rural physician education. Linda was working at the clinic serving as the education coordinator for the Baraboo residency. Jenny was age 24, had graduated from the UW–Madison, was working as a school psychologist, and was planning a master's degree in school psychology through the UW–Whitewater. Finally, Tim was age 21 and was a junior at the University of Wisconsin–Stevens Point studying communications/journalism.

Several doctors in our county had organized the "Haiti Medical Mission of Wisconsin" partnering with the rural village of Thiotte, Haiti to offer healthcare. Tim and I volunteered to go on one of these two-week missions.

❧

We had just gotten off the plane in Port-au-Prince, Haiti. We headed to the airport terminal to pick up our baggage, which included medical supplies as well as our clothes. As we entered the Haiti airport terminal, we were warned to not let anyone volunteer to carry our luggage for us, because we might never see it again.

At the main terminal, a mob of people immediately surrounded us, motioning to carry our luggage. One man, paralyzed from the waist down, was not on crutches or in a wheelchair but walked on his calloused hands. His clothes looked like rags. He begged for anything he could secure. It was sad to see this.

We arrived at the baggage area and picked up our bags then went through customs without much of a problem.

At one point, a man in an army uniform asked me in a stern voice, "What is in those bags you are carrying?"

I had medical supplies in the pockets. Before I had a chance to say anything, one of the more experienced Haiti travelers behind me yelled out, "Bibles!" and the guard let us go through. Medical supplies might have been confiscated while Bibles would not.

Finally, through the terminal, we boarded several jeeps driven by the guides and interpreters for our group. We loaded our baggage into the vehicles, and off we drove to a halfway house in Port-Au Prince to spend the first night.

The drive over to the halfway house was eye-opening. I saw skinny dogs running around, people cooking on the sidewalks over small charcoal burners, dilapidated housing, handicapped people navigating without disability aids, and children playing naked in flooded streets.

Our guide, Lamont, asked, "What is your first impression of Haiti?"

"I am saddened at what I see," I said.

"You are in the good part of town," Lamont replied.

At the halfway house, the former Catholic priest who runs it greeted us happily.

After unloading the jeeps and filing away our luggage, the next stop was a visit to Mother Theresa's house. We were driven to a building where several Catholic nuns worked with ill or abandoned children. Some were very dehydrated from diarrhea, and the sisters were feeding them and/or giving them IV fluids.

Tim walked into a room where he was surrounded by young children hanging on his arms and body. They apparently were starved for love and attention. Tim sat down in a rocking chair and immediately had five to six children on his lap. As I watched Tim with a grin on his face and children fighting for position on his lap, a nun walked into the room.

Tim asked, "What are these children being treated for?"

The sister replied, "These children are being treated for tuberculosis."

With a surprised look on his face, Tim stood up abruptly and excused himself.

After touring Mother Theresa's, we returned to the halfway house. We ate dinner there and afterward retired outside for socialization.

Outside, a group of Haitians played basketball. Since Tim played in high school, he went down to the court to

see if he could get into the game. After just a few minutes, one of the teams invited him to join. Following a
few passes up and down the court, Tim finally scored a
basket. At that moment, the other nine players on the
court stopped and gave him a round of applause in a
friendly, supportive way. They accepted him, the only
Caucasian, into the game as a friend. It was a lovely gesture. What if the world could be like this? We learned
that even though Haitians are some of the poorest people on earth, they seemed friendly and accepting.

We slept at the halfway house that night. The following morning after breakfast, we loaded into the jeeps
and headed to the mountains toward the small town
of Thiotte. The distance from Port-au-Prince to Thiotte is 109 km or about 68 miles. It took us three and
a half hours to drive this distance through the winding, mountainous roads with large potholes. The warm,
humid weather made the trip all that more strenuous.

We finally arrived in Thiotte and unpacked our bags
at the Catholic church. Several cots were set up in a
room at the back of the church, where we were to sleep
and leave our luggage. A small, filthy bathroom off this
back room had feces on the floor, a toilet that barely
flushed, and a showerhead that produced only a tiny
stream of water for bathing. We were warned to wear
sandals while in the bathroom and to not worry if we
can't flush the toilet.

We freshened up from our trip the best we could.
There would be a church service in our honor within
the next hour, as a sort of greeting by the village. The

people seemed remarkably friendly and happy, despite how deprived they are.

A group of children from the village began to follow us around. One child named James connected with me since we had the same name. James asked me for things like a pen to write with or a ball to bounce around. Apparently, these were gifts that had been handed out to the children in the past. These simple items are taken for granted in America, but they brought such delight to Haitian children.

For the church service, we sat on chairs at the back of the altar. The priest began a traditional Catholic ceremony. Halfway through the service, he stopped and said something in Creole to the congregation. A children's choir began to sing a beautiful piece of music. These kids sounded like professionals.

At that moment, a long line formed outside the church. While the children sang, people danced up the center aisle of the church, each one with a gift for us.

We were instructed to form a line, and one by one each of us met these people at the front of the altar to receive the gifts.

The children continued to sing as we received such gifts as chickens, lambs, feathered ornaments, fruit, and other items. One elderly lady wore an old-time hat with a flower on a stem. She carried a small purse with her. When I greeted her at the altar, she fumbled with the zipper of this small, dime-store-type bag. She finally unzipped it and proudly handed me an egg. She walked away with a satisfied smile on her face. It was touching.

This line of people bearing gifts went on for about forty-five minutes, a very moving and spiritual experience. We placed most of the donations behind the altar. The church service ended, and we had some snacks and retired for the night. It was a long day.

The following morning, I woke up to two dogs fighting out back in the courtyard of the church. Apparently, some of the animal gifts presented to us had been sacrificed, and the dogs were fighting over the remains.

We gathered for breakfast. A woman said, "I want you to all join hands now. A Haitian song will be sung before we eat." The members of our team who had been on this trip before were familiar with the words to the song. Tim and I hummed along.

The food was excellent, and we thanked the staff for their work in preparing the meal. We headed off to conduct our first clinic in the church.

Out in the courtyard of the church, a large crowd of people gathered. A nurse circulated through the crowd, triaging medical problems and handing people numbers that represented what order they were to be seen by the doctors inside. Some of the people were quite theatrical, faking a fainting episode, or groaning in pain, trying to get a lower number.

One of the first Haitians I saw was a young woman brought in by her family. Through the interpreter, I was told, "They claim that she is pregnant and has delivered the afterbirth first. The baby is still inside her."

She laid on a cot in the courtyard outside in a pool of blood. I went out to see her only to find they had mistaken a macerated baby for the placenta. At probably around six months pregnant, she, unfortunately, delivered a nonviable infant. A fragile umbilical cord the size of a small pencil protruded outside of her vagina.

I asked that she be brought into the church so I could examine her further in private, but the cathedral was full. A nurse brought me gloves and suggested I inspect her on the cot. She tried to erect a barrier of sheets tied to poles around us for some privacy. I pulled gently on this thin cord to deliver the real placenta, but I feared I might break it, leaving the placenta up inside of her. This was all done on the cot, in the courtyard outside, not a very sterile environment. A crowd gathered around us, looking over the barrier to watch me, and one of the nurses came over to disperse them.

"Why don't we start an IV on this young lady and I am going to use some Pitocin (a hormone that causes uterine contractions) to see if I can get the placenta delivered," I said.

After a few hours, the placenta was visible at the cervix. I again gently pulled on the umbilical cord, but I felt it begin to tear. So as not to cause further tearing of the cord, I reached up inside this poor woman and did a manual removal of the small placenta. Because this was all done outside under what I considered decidedly nonsterile conditions, I asked if we had any antibiotics. I was told there are intravenous penicillin and amoxicillin available. I gave a dose of IV penicillin, and because she wanted to go home immediately, I gave her amoxicillin tablets to take with her with instructions on its use. We observed her for 20–30 minutes after her IV penicillin dose to make sure there was no allergic reaction. She then got up off the cot and left the courtyard on her own. She walked to her home a few blocks away.

The next day, I made a house call on her and found her working around her home, carrying water up from the stream and cooking. She had no fever, no abdominal pain, and no malodorous vaginal drainage. She was taking the amoxicillin as prescribed. She acted as if nothing had happened. I wondered if something like this had happened to her before.

The first day of seeing Haitians was eye-opening. I was struck by the severity of the cases. One man was brought into the clinic because he had a "sore on his forehead." He was an elderly man who looked about seventy to eighty years old but may have been much younger. Most people had no idea how old they were as there were no birth certificates.

What I saw was skin cancer that had eroded into his skull, and the frontal lobe of his brain was showing. We could not do much for him. This would require major surgery. We gave the family some pain medication and told them there was not much we could do and that he was dying. The smell was awful. The nurse washed up as much of the wound as she could, wrapped his head in a bandage, and taught the family how to change the dressing daily. We gave them some dressing material and pain tablets to take home.

One of the medical students tapped me on the shoulder. "I have a young boy about age eight or ten brought in by his mother. His abdomen is huge, and he is having trouble breathing. Can you look at him with me?"

The medical student remembered him from a previous visit that she made a year ago to Haiti. She said at that time, they had diagnosed him with probable rheumatic fever and Sydenham's chorea. This is a condition that results from a strep infection, where the patient develops jerking movements that look like twitches. Patients with rheumatic fever may develop arthritis, nodules beneath the skin, a heart murmur, and a rash.

I listened to this boy's heart and heard a heart murmur called mitral stenosis (first heart sound, opening snap, followed by a diastolic rumble heart murmur). This probably ten-year-old boy was in congestive heart failure from mitral valve heart disease. The large abdomen appeared to be ascites (fluid collection in his belly). He had massive swelling of his ankles all the way up to his knees. He suffered from advanced heart failure.

We gave this boy a medication called Lasix, a diuretic. Over the next several hours, he began to urinate in massive amounts. We decided to give him some oral potassium and more Lasix. We had no laboratory to follow his electrolytes. We made room for him to stay overnight in the church. His delighted mother saw him begin to lose weight and breathe easier. She had tears of joy in her eyes. Her son had improved. To her, we were miracle workers.

One of the other doctors and I were told that there was a cardiac surgeon in the United States who would evaluate and possibly operate on people from Haiti free of charge. We decided to purchase an echocardiogram for this patient, which could be done in Port-au-Prince. We would have the echocardiogram sent to us in the United States, and if it showed mitral stenosis, we would contact this cardiac surgeon.

While we treated this young boy with congestive heart failure, another case arrived. A mother and father brought in their daughter, who appeared to be a young teenager. The parents spoke anxiously in Creole.

The interpreter said, "They say she has become stiff in all her muscles. She is having difficulty walking, speaking, and swallowing."

On exam, her blood pressure was slightly elevated, at 160/95. She had stiff muscles that were painful during a range of motion. She was unable to open her mouth completely. Further history revealed that she had stepped on a nail in the recent past. Her foot had been sore for several days, and it turned red around the puncture.

I had never seen a case of this before but had read about "lockjaw," or tetanus, in my medical school studies. We don't see tetanus in the United States because of our immunization programs. Immunizations are practically nonexistent in Haitians. The bacteria causing "lockjaw" is Clostridium tetani. This germ secretes a toxin that causes these effects on muscles. The bacteria contaminate wounds and are found in soil or in the gastrointestinal tract of animals.

Today's treatment for tetanus is directed toward stopping toxin production with antibiotics, neutralizing toxin effects with vaccines, and controlling muscle spasms. We needed to provide tetanus immune globulin as well as active immunization with tetanus toxoid. The antimicrobial used is called metronidazole, which is given intravenously. We did not have intravenous metronidazole with us, nor did we have any vaccines. But we did have intravenous penicillin. We decided to treat this young lady with penicillin in hopes that this would help. We had Valium to give her for her muscle spasms. We washed the wound and applied local treatment. The family chose to stay in the church overnight.

While we started her IV and double-checked on the boy with congestive heart failure, a young girl came in on a donkey. Those with her said she has been in labor for three days. She had been unable to deliver the baby. She had not been hemorrhaging.

I examined her vaginally, and I found the baby's head to be in an occiput posterior position (sunny side up, or the baby looking at the ceiling). She had a lot of back pain. She appeared exhausted, and her pushing with contractions was less than optimal after an alleged three days. We did not have a vacuum unit for me to apply to the head and attempt to deliver the baby with instruments. We found a pair of mismatched forceps, but I thought it would be dangerous to try to use them. I, therefore, decided to try manually rotating the baby's head with my hand. This was not usually that successful for me, but for some reason, it worked that day.

Just as I started having her push after having rotated the head, a group of women showed up from her village. They kicked us all out and began managing her labor themselves. Every time she had a contraction, two women on each leg held her legs out and slapped her inner thighs repeatedly with their hands until the uterine contraction was over. When she felt more comfortable, they fed her beer. We tried to negotiate with the women in Creole, but they did not listen to us. They planned to manage this labor themselves.

After several more contractions and probably a total of two beers, she finally delivered the baby. Of course, the baby appeared intoxicated, floppy, and did not breathe right away. At that point, the women turned the case over to us, and we used an Ambu bag to ventilate the baby while we stimulated the baby to get some response. After several minutes, the baby let out a cry, and everyone cheered. One of the other doctors attended to the baby, and I turned my attention to mom and proceeded to deliver the placenta.

As soon as the baby was stable, and mom's placenta was surrendered, mom and baby boarded the donkey and left. The lay midwives thanked us in Creole and went with her.

The rest of that day we saw young children who had been dressed up by their parents for the doctor visit. Most of them just wanted a physical examination and some vitamins. Sometimes they wanted medication for worms that had been noted in the child's stool. I probably saw fifty to seventy-five men, women, and children that day.

It was quite rewarding compared to practicing medicine in the U.S. We saved time and could see many more patients because we did not have to spend a lot of time documenting for legal purposes in case of a lawsuit. We saw the patient, and the only things we recorded on our laptop computer were the diagnosis and the treatment rendered.

My son's job throughout the day was working in the pharmacy with the pharmacist, Sue, who had accompanied us on the trip. Tim started up a medical record system that included each patient's medications on a laptop computer.

Tim enjoyed interacting with the pharmacist and the University of Wisconsin pharmacy student who had volunteered for the Haiti medical mission. Tim became an asset to the team, and I was very proud to see my son responsibly helping others. His sense of empathy and caring had been evident during his sister's illness when Jenny was being treated for cancer. He brought these positive traits to Haiti with him. He became quite popular with the Haitian children in this small village as he played soccer and basketball with them.

The day ended at five p.m., although there were still plenty of people in the courtyard of the church. They were told to come back the next day. The nursing staff and interpreters were protecting us.

We double-checked our patient with tetanus and our patient with congestive heart failure, who appeared to be stable. All the medical personnel then gathered on the roof of the church to decompress and to discuss the cases we had seen during the daytime. There was a Haitian radio station broadcasting across the courtyard, and we listened to some great music.

After dinner, it was quite easy to retire as we were exhausted. I wondered what would come the next day.

The following morning, we went to check on our children with congestive heart failure and tetanus. They were both doing very well. The little boy with congestive heart failure was amazed at how well he could breathe. He decided to go to Port-au-Prince for the echocardiogram that we had agreed to purchase for him. If he had mitral stenosis from rheumatic fever, he might need cardiac surgery, although I was skeptical this could be done with his later-stage disease. We provided his mother with some Lasix to give him daily. Since we were unable to check his kidney function and electrolytes before putting him on this medication, we went with a smaller dose.

The girl with tetanus was also much improved. She felt that her muscles were more limber and did not ache like they did before. She was a bit sedated on the Valium. Her swallowing was recovering, and she could talk much better. The family felt it was time for her to leave. We tried to convince them to stay to receive further doses of her IV penicillin and to monitor her further. They disagreed, feeling she was much improved and thanked us. There was no stopping them. We gave them oral penicillin and wished them well.

The rest of the morning we saw many cases late in their disease evolution. We saw several instances of what we thought was likely HIV/AIDS, a septic child, several skin infections, some headaches and neck pain, and the usual request for vitamins and worm medication.

We did run a few IVs on people who had diarrhea and appeared dehydrated.

After lunch, Lamont came up to me and said, "Would you like to see where the people get their water and why you saw so many cases of diarrhea, headaches, and neck pain?"

I said, "Sure I would."

He took us to a steep hill. At the bottom of this slope was a stream, where we saw many Haitians washing their clothes. The women would scoop the water up in large containers, place them on top of their heads, balance these cylinders, and walk back up this rather steep hill. Lamont told us it was quite tricky to get the people to believe in "germ theory." Many people would bring the water back up to their huts and begin drinking and cooking with it. The medical teams were trying to get them to boil the water first, but the Haitians did not understand why.

As we began walking back up the hill, I heard a woman speaking in Creole behind me. She appeared impatient with me and spoke in a rather stern voice. She carried a large container of water on her head.

Lamont began to laugh. "What are you laughing at, Lamont?" I said while stepping aside to let her pass us.

As she went by, I noted she was about eight months pregnant and balanced probably five gallons of water on her head (forty pounds). Now I understood diarrhea, neck pain, and headaches in the patients I had been seeing.

Several days went by seeing the same types of cases over and over. These included headaches, neck pain, diarrhea, worms, rashes, large hydroceles and hernias on men, and many young children who requested a physical exam and vitamins. Of course, none of them had ever had immunizations.

One evening after dinner, someone came running into the church, calling for the doctors.

"There has been a serious accident a few miles from the church. A large two-level bus, a tap-tap, was taking people down to Port-au-Prince for shopping. The overloaded coach went around the corner in the mountains, and it tipped and rolled down the hill. There were many people injured, and medical personnel is needed immediately."

One of the women at the church advised us to be careful. "You will be going into the forest where a Catholic priest was once robbed and shot. This could be a dangerous mission."

After a brief group discussion, we concluded we couldn't ignore injured people that we might be able to help. Several of the doctors, including myself, as well as several nurses, jumped into two jeeps, and we headed for the accident.

As I was leaving, Tim yelled, "Please be careful, Dad."

By the time we arrived, it was pitch dark. As we approached the area of the crash, we saw a bonfire. Some of the Haitians had taken the tires off the bus and started a fire for warmth. It was beginning to rain and get cold. I will never forget the sight of the overturned bus on the side of the hill and a hillside filled with bodies.

We went from body to body, looking for life. We came upon one young man who was moaning. A quick assessment showed he had multiple extremity injuries, a chest injury, a faint pulse, and he was in shock.

"Let's get two IV's going on him with normal saline. How about some morphine. He looks like he's in pain. We will need to immobilize his neck," I said.

After our team completed all these things, we placed him on a large piece of plywood in the back of a pickup truck in Trendelenburg (feet elevated above his head so that blood would flow to the head and heart). A man agreed to drive this make-shift ambulance to Port-Au-Prince, where there was a hospital. As I saw this person leave in the back of the vehicle, a torrential downpour of cold rain began. I felt almost sure that he would never make it. It was likely a three- to four-hour drive to Port-Au-Prince at night in the rain down a mountainside road with huge potholes.

We continued to go from dead body to dead body and finally found a second man moaning. He too was unconscious, had a very faint pulse, no discernible blood pressure, and appeared to have massive head and chest injuries. There was no other vehicle now to transport him to any hospital. He seemed to have multiple fractures involving his lower extremities.

"What do you think?" I said to the team.

Dr. Brian, the ER physician, said, "This man is in pain and is suffering. There is no ambulance or even a vehicle to take him anywhere. He is going to die."

"I agree," I said as I tried to see through my glasses in the rain. All of us were drenched and cold from the downfall.

I thought back to the principle of "*double effect.*" This principle says it is permissible to risk harm such as the death of a human being as a side effect to promoting good (relief of pain, in this case with morphine). I recalled my patient who was dying of cancer on her couch. I remember giving her extra morphine to alleviate her agitation and possible pain she was experiencing. The situation we now confronted was no different.

Dr. Brian, a nurse, and I came to the decision that the best thing for this patient would be a standard dose of morphine and more if needed. The fact that he continued to moan indicated to us that he was likely in a lot of pain.

We tried giving him this dose of morphine in the arm, in the groin, a hand, and the foot but couldn't find a vein. Intramuscular morphine given to a patient in shock would not be that effective. I finally gave the morphine intracardiac (straight into the heart). As I gave him the medication, he stopped breathing. He had died. Perhaps the morphine caused him to stop breathing. It was also plausible he died of his other injuries, but I still felt anxious that I had just committed euthanasia. My colleagues thought we had done the humane thing for him.

The rain increased. We were thoroughly soaked and cold. Bodies covered the side of the hill. We examined each one of them and could not find anyone else alive.

I could hardly see through my glasses. Several of the Haitians by the overturned bus encouraged us to go back to the church. They thanked us for our work. We later heard that the man we sent to Port-au-Prince in the pickup truck had lived.

I slept fitfully that night. I kept questioning the doctrine of "*double effect,*" but in the end, I felt more confident we did the right thing, considering the circumstances.

The next day, we arose for breakfast and started seeing patients again. I noted a man in the courtyard who had been there every day, waiting to be examined by the doctors. Being shy and less aggressive, he never seemed to get a number to be seen by the doctor. I pointed him out to one of the clinic staff.

Two more days went by, and it was our last day in Haiti. The crowds had thinned. Once again, I saw the shy man standing against a fence in the courtyard. I pointed him out to the staff, and he was brought over to me to be seen. The staff member told me he lived two hours away from the church and that he had walked to the church to be seen every day for the two weeks we had been there. When he was not seen, he walked home only to return the next day hoping to see a doctor.

Through the interpreter, I asked him, "Can you tell me what you would like me to look at?" He pulled his pants down and showed me a large inguinal hernia that he had been walking with four hours each day to and from the clinic.

The general surgeon, Dr. Tony, had been doing hernia and hydrocele operations all week using local anesthesia. Our patient finally went under the knife.

After getting his hernia fixed, he had a radiant smile on his face. He got up off the table and began his walk home, just as he had done the previous days.

At the end of our Haiti trip, it took me several weeks to decompress from the experience after I returned home.

ॐ

My first day back to work in the United States produced an unusual rural patient. He wore a suit and tie and looked to be in his fifties.

"Doctor, you are twenty minutes late for this appointment," he said to me. "My time is just as valuable as yours. You need to be on time with your patients. For what you charge for these visits, I expect better service."

I apologized saying, "You are justified with your anger. I am behind. I am so sorry. What can I do to help you today?"

He told me about the severe cold he has had for three days. "Doctor, I am leaving on a business trip, and I need to get rid of this ASAP. I can't be sick and miss this meeting. I need antibiotics."

After examining him, I informed him this was likely a viral illness and antibiotics were not indicated at this time. I talked with him about conservative treatment and flying with respiratory congestion. I gave him warning signs on when to seek care again. He left unhappy with me that I did not wave the magic wand and instantly cure him.

This man's behavior was hard to take after what I had observed in Haiti. I realized this patient was atypical but it still bothered me.

For several weeks, I kept contrasting in my mind this person with Haitians. Those in Haiti have minimal healthcare but were so appreciative of anything we could do for them. It was hard to come back and begin documenting detailed notes on every move I made to avoid potential malpractice. This contrasts with the much shorter medical progress notes when seeing patients in Haiti, where I could also see a higher volume of patients. My concise medical progress notes in Haiti would not pass the test in an American courtroom.

I finally decompressed, but I still couldn't get out of my mind the extent of illness I had seen in Haiti. I could not forget the man I gave the dose of morphine to on the side of that hill in the rain, thinking he would never make it three to four hours to Port-au-Prince. The broad medical knowledge base required of a primary care physician I found most useful in Haiti.

This was an unforgettable experience, giving me the highest respect for Haitians. About a month after returning from Haiti, we received the echocardiogram on the ten-year-old boy. Indeed, it showed mitral stenosis (a damaged heart valve causing his congestive heart failure). The cardiac surgeon agreed to see this boy in the United States. We were unable, however, to find the mother and her son when we contacted the Catholic Church in Thiotte. They suspected the boy had died.

Chapter 26

Why Us?

MY DAUGHTER CALLED ME THIS AFTERNOON. "Dad, have you noticed mom being forgetful? I have noted that she asks me the same questions over and over. I am concerned."

While in Madison, Linda had completed her master's degree in public policy and healthcare administration. In Baraboo, she had taken the job of education coordinator at the University of Wisconsin–Baraboo Rural Physician Training program. Linda assisted the residents in getting their rotations completed. She ran the recruitment program for prospective applicants and shared in the work to keep the program in compliance with the national residency review commission.

I too noticed that Linda's prior superb education coordinator duties had become more challenging for her.

Linda had been talking about retiring. I suspected she was noting increasing problems with organization. We had some discussions at home, and we finally decided it was time for her to retire. She requested no fanfare. I sensed Linda felt somewhat embarrassed by her increasing difficulty with the job. She had previously been so organized. Our residency program always passed our national reviews with flying colors. The education coordinator plays a vital role in this appraisal.

It wasn't long after retirement that she became quite bored at home. This was not her. I started wondering whether she had "retirement depression." She had always been a very active person, never sitting down. She was either working on a home project, outside gardening or taking care of our flower beds around the house. She was active in a neighborhood book club, attended the Merrimac Community Women's Club, and went to an exercise class with a group from the neighborhood once weekly. For a while, she got up at five-thirty every morning to participate in a swimming exercise class at the high school with another group of friends. She was a kayaker and had taken weekend trips around the state of Wisconsin with several of her friends. It was very unusual for her to tell me she was bored.

We decided together for her to see her doctor and have a physical examination. She related her boredom and her memory disorder to her physician. Proper workup ensued, including blood testing, brain imaging, and finally a few months later specialty consultation. She was sent for neuropsychiatric testing which lasted for five hours one day.

All this testing revealed what I did not want to hear: Linda had early Alzheimer's disease.

We had so much looked forward to an active retirement. I too was thinking about retirement, having recruited one of our previous residency graduates to come back to direct the Baraboo rural physician training program. I planned to serve as assistant program director to break him into the job. Alzheimer's disease was going to alter our plans.

I could see the effects this had on Linda. The radiant smile I fell in love with during our college chemistry class was disappearing. She became frustrated when she couldn't remember something. She had been valedictorian of her high school class and an honor student at the University of Illinois–Urbana. She had excelled in pharmacy school and in her master's program at the University of Wisconsin–Madison.

Since her diagnosis, Linda had the usual progression one would expect with Alzheimer's disease. She was treated with donepezil (Aricept) and later a combination of donepezil (Aricept) and memantine (Namenda). Initially, she had problems coming up with the right word and difficulty remembering recent events. She had increasing issues with planning and organizing. Later, she required increasing care of her daily activities. Such things as dressing, bathing, toileting, transfers, and language became increasing challenges for her. She had visual-spatial difficulties when she walked. I became a full-time caregiver.

I experienced, first hand as a caregiver and not a doctor, how our healthcare system deals with chronic debilitating medical problems. Although Linda and I had assistance from a home health agency, long-term care insurance, and hospice, I discovered how difficult it is to navigate our healthcare system in America. We had three nurse practitioners visiting us quarterly to fill out progress reports and to update care plans on Linda for their respective agencies. They all duplicated what the others had done. It was not their fault. They were doing their jobs, but these organizations were not connected. One nurse could have collected the information and shared it with the others.

It was expensive. Dealing with the billing through our long-term care insurance company was challenging to begin with and took months to straighten out. Our home health assistance was caring, kind, and competent but we experienced a turnover of certified nursing assistants helping us as they moved on to new jobs. This turnover can confuse someone with cognitive impairment. Turnover caused me to duplicate a review of our home procedures to new personnel as they changed over.

As I dealt with corporate insurance companies with Part B supplements and Part D drug plans, I attempted to chat with someone online about a question only to get a message: "*You currently are in the queue. A chat specialist will be with you shortly.*" Thirty minutes later I gave up. If I tried to ask my question through a phone call, I would encounter a long menu of choices before finally talking to someone from another state who had no idea who I was. Refills for prescriptions could be a nightmare dealing with a large national organization. The local town pharmacy was much more comfortable and more personal to deal with. The paperwork I had to fill out was vast, duplicative, and repetitive.

The most comfortable system for me to deal with was Medicare and the Medicare Hospice benefit for palliative care. It was a walk in the park. The primary focus was on health, not on getting your bill paid. The only downside to Medicare was it did not cover assisted living, memory center care, or nursing home care (long-term care). This would have to be funded by our own personal finances or one's long-term care coverage. The cost of long-term care admission to a facility in our area ranged between $150–$350 per day. Most people cannot afford these prices or afford premiums for long-term care insurance. Just think of the money we could save nationwide getting rid of duplication and paperwork in our system (administrative costs) and having one affordable system to deal with whether it be private, public, or a hybrid.

I am no expert, but perhaps Medicare for all could cover hospital care, and the private insurance industry could cover outpatient care. It is hospital and long-term care that can bankrupt someone. Outpatient care is less expensive. Our insurance industry would remain in business with more affordable premiums if they covered only outpatient care. Our health science in the United States is superb but navigating our complex healthcare system can be rough, duplicative, costly, and impersonal for many. I had first-hand experience.

I also ponder whether a program like the St. Jude or Shriners hospital programs for children could be developed for the other end of the age spectrum, seniors.

Unless one is exceptionally wealthy, long-term care can abolish the average couple's life savings like a massive hospital bill.

Financial donations spirited by captivating marketing programs for St. Jude and the Shriners hospitals help families who are facing childhood cancer and other disability. Their TV commercials are very touching. Maybe we could develop an "Aging America Program." I know Americans are amongst the most generous people in the world. The "Aging America Program" could be marketed on TV with commercials like St. Jude or the Shriners to help cover long-term care costs. These TV ads would be much more pleasant to see compared to the numerous drug commercials that feature the most expensive drugs that seem to dominate TV commercials.

This "Aging America Program" might help people afford home care, assisted living, memory care, and nursing home care which are all poorly funded in our current system. Through donations from national marketing, the two ends of the age spectrum, young and old, would be better covered.

≈♠

As a caregiver, I see my role as trying to make Linda's life in retirement as rewarding as possible, given the challenges we both are facing. We have been through tough times before (childhood cancer, medical school, and residency). It doesn't seem fair, but those are the cards handed to us. Like the Catholic nun said when our daughter, Jenny, was admitted with her Wilms tumor and I asked her why a God would give a child cancer: "I don't know why this happened to you. God works in mysterious ways."

We have much to be thankful for. We try to focus on the positive. Linda put her heart and soul into Jenny and Tim's care in the early chemotherapy days. Years later, Jenny delivered two children. Our second grandchild (Aleyna Linn) was born on Linda's birthday. What a gift as payback.

After Jenny's chemotherapy, radiation, and surgery were completed, our family withstood six years of follow-up wondering with each doctor visit whether Jenny's cancer would recur. All of Jenny's follow-ups were favorable. Jenny is enjoying raising her kids and serving as a school psychologist. She has a very supportive group of friends. Our grandchildren are treasures in our lives.

Our son, Tim, is a wonderful man who remains very involved with the family. He has received many journalism awards and loves writing.

I have endured fourteen years of childhood cancer and Alzheimer's disease in our family. I feel a sense of accomplishment believing I balanced being a husband, father, grandfather, and a doctor successfully during these fourteen years of hard times. I am thankful to have been a family physician having had the opportunity to become involved in so many people's lives while I attempted to help them.

At the time of this writing, Linda is in year eight of her Alzheimer's disease. Although she has lost a significant amount of function, she has had no behavior problems or wandering to date. The home care and hospice personnel comment that she is kind and easy to care for.

We are thankful for all our former colleagues; and, of course, our immediate and extended families. We are grateful to our friends, our neighborhoods, and our church. These connections have been so important to us.

A recent example exemplifies this. One day our doorbell rang. When I answered, it was Dr. Brent, the Pediatric allergist, his wife Cathy, and Scott who had played football in the NFL and his family. We had not seen Scott in probably twenty-five years although we had followed his career on TV. My heart warmed as they all greeted me with hugs at the door.

Scott immediately went to the couch where Linda sat. He took Linda's hand. "Hi, Linda. I wanted to come to see someone who meant a lot to me when I was growing up; almost like a second mom."

Alzheimer's disease had stolen Linda's language, but I know seeing Scott and his family meant a lot to her. Linda had a smile on her face and was in such a good mood for the rest of the afternoon. Caregivers notice these subtleties.

I too owe it to Linda. Without Linda, I would never have made it this far, considering my background. My parents could not afford medical school. They were barely able to assist me with my undergraduate education although they certainly tried. Linda was a gift to my life. At the time of this writing, we are going on forty-nine years of marriage.

I know I will eventually have to confront the end. Alzheimer's disease is currently incurable. Will I care for her at home with hospice or will I need to move Linda to a nursing home, memory care unit, or inpatient hospice unit? How will we close the last chapter of our life together? This is unknown.

Bibliography

AARP 2015 [National Alliance for Caregiving and AARP. (2015). Caregiving in the U.S.]

Claire K. Ankuda, MD, MPH, Stephen M. Petterson, Ph.D., Peter Wingrove, BS and Andrew W. Bazemore, MD, MPH. 2017 Jan; 15(1). "Regional Variation in Primary Care Involvement at the End of Life." *Annals of Family Medicine* 63-67. Accessed January 25, 2018. http://www.annfammed.org/content/15/1/63.

Dieleman JL1, Squires E1, Bui AL2, Campbell M, Chapin A, Hamavid H, Horst C, Li Z, Matyasz T, Reynolds A, Sadat N, Schneider MT, Murray CJL. 2017. "Factors Associated With Increases in US Healthcare Spending." *JAMA* 1668–1678.

Gerald Friedman, Ph.D. 2013. *The Expanded and Improved Medicare for All Act: How we can afford a national single-payer health plan.* Executive Summary, Funding HR 676.

Maron, Dina Fine. 2017. "Maternal Health Care Is Disappearing in Rural America." *Scientific American*, February 15: https://www.scientificamerican.com/article/maternal -health-care-is-disappearing-in-rural-america/.

National Rural Health Association. 2017. *About Rural Health Care.* December 16. Accessed January 25, 2018. https://www.ruralhealthweb.org/about-nrha/about-rural-health-care.

—. November 2006. Issue Paper, "Recruitment and Retention of a Quality Health Work Force in Rural Areas, Number 4: Oral Health."

PACE. 2017. *(ALSO) Advanced Life Support in Obstetrics.* Accessed January 25, 2018. https://www.centro-pace.org/en/programs/advanced-life-support-in-obstetrics-also/.

Peiyin Hung, MSPH, Katy B. Kozhimannil, Ph.D., Michelle M. Casey, MS, Carrie Henning-Smith, Ph.D., Shailendra Prasad, MBBS, MPH. 2016. *State Variations in the Rural Obstetric Workforce.* Policy Brief, Minneapolis: University of Minnesota Rural Health Research Center.

Robyn Latessa, MD, and Lisa Ray, MD. 2005 Mar;12(3). "Should You Treat Yourself, Family or Friends?" *Family Practice Management* 41–44.

ScholarshipStats.com. 2016–2017. *Odds of a High School Athlete Playing in College.* Accessed January 25, 2018. http://www.scholarshipstats.com/varsityodds.html.

Shakespeare, William, Jay L. Halio (Editor). 2008. *The Merchant of Venice: The Oxford Shakespeare The Merchant of Venice (Oxford World's Classics) 1st Edition.* Oxford University Press.

TS Nesbitt, E H Larson, R A Rosenblatt, and L G Hart. 1997. "Access to maternity care in rural Washington: Its effect on neonatal outcomes and resource use." *American Journal of Public Health (AJPH)* 85–90.

Acknowledgments

DR. ROBERT KOTTKAMP IS PROFESSOR EMERI-
tus of Educational Leadership and Policy Studies,
Hofstra University. He has co-authored six books and
supervised many doctoral dissertations. Dr. Kottkamp
proved to be a tremendous help to me with this book.
Bob and his wife, Ginny, have greatly influenced our
lives during our times of transition.

Mrs. Kay Johnston is a retired English teacher and
former Teacher of the Year at Belleville high school in
Belleville, Wisconsin. She has taught high school English in several Wisconsin school districts, and she too
was a tremendous help in creating this book. Kay Johnston and her husband, Dave, and their family have posi-
tively influenced us in so many ways. To this day, our
families remain the best of friends.

One final acknowledgment goes to what I consider
an exceptional movie that made such an impact on my
family and especially Linda and me. In 1989, Phil Alden
Robinson directed the movie *Field of Dreams* starring
Kevin Costner, Amy Madigan, James Earl Jones, Ray
Liotta, and Burt Lancaster. To this day, my family has
often referred to this movie by occasionally kidding

me calling me "Moonlight Graham." Even now thirty years later, my wife Linda will cry during the last scenes of this touching movie when Ray Kinsella says to his estranged father, "Dad, you want to have a catch?" Our family has visited Dyersville, Iowa where the movie was filmed. (yes, people will come).

In the movie, Burt Lancaster plays Dr. Archibald Wright "Moonlight" Graham, a small-town generalist physician who played baseball and had dreamed of being a major league baseball player (a true story). As the story goes, after playing ball at the University of North Carolina at Chapel Hill, Archie Graham went on to play class B and C baseball in the minor leagues for seven seasons. He hit .272 in 108 games for Manchester in 1904 and was later purchased by the New York Giants joining them on May 23, 1905. On June 29th, 1905 "Archie" got into his first major league baseball game in the eighth inning. In the top of the ninth, he was on deck to bat when the inning ended with the third out and he unfortunately never got to bat. He played right field in the bottom of the ninth but never had a ball hit to him.

Archie Graham never got into a game after that. A medical career followed, and after reading an ad listing an opening for a doctor in Minnesota, Doc Graham journeyed to the small town of Chisholm, Minnesota, accepted the job, and never left. He practiced there until his death in 1965—fifty-four years later.

Ray Kinsella in the movie (played by Kevin Costner) thought it was a tragedy that Moonlight Graham never got the opportunity to play major league baseball, to which Doc Graham replied:

> "Son, if I'd only been a doctor for five minutes, now that would have been a tragedy."

I agree with Doc Graham. Burt Lancaster was one of my favorite actors when I was growing up. I can relate to Doc Graham because I shared similar small-town doctor-patient experiences that he likely had. I also played baseball through the years as a shortstop and second baseman. I played peanut league, little league, pony league, American Legion ball, Chicago shoreline ball, high school ball, and I did a very brief stint at college ball. I had an opportunity to play semi-pro ball one summer for nominal pay. Even though I longed to be in the major leagues, I knew I was not good enough. I had gone as far as I was going to go in baseball. Instead, my path in life also took me to medical school. Like Doc Graham, I too feel it would have been a tragedy to have been a family physician for only five minutes.

Doc Graham was dedicated, kind, and a pillar of the community. In *Field of Dreams,* the townspeople commented, "No child in need in the community was without eyeglasses, milk, clothing, or a ticket to the ballgame."

What a silent hero. I know there are many doctors like him all over America in small towns. It is obvious why I connected with this movie, why my kids tease me, and why Linda gets emotional during the last scene. This style of medicine focusing on dreams, caring, long-term relationships, and kindness, as well as the spiritual theme throughout the movie, has served as an inspiration for me through the years. Thank you to Hollywood for touching us so profoundly.

About the Author

FAMILY PHYSICIAN DR. JAMES DAMOS HAS EARNED a reputation for storytelling among medical students, interns, residents, physician colleagues, and the lay public. He has received local, state, national, and international recognition during his career. His medical career spans rural, urban, academic, and private practice.

With the help of his colleagues and the American Academy of Family Physicians, he participated in the development of the now international Advanced Life Support in Obstetrics (ALSO) provider and instructor courses. He and his colleagues developed the University of Wisconsin–Baraboo Rural Physician Training Program that is now nationally recognized. Both projects focused on rural access to healthcare.

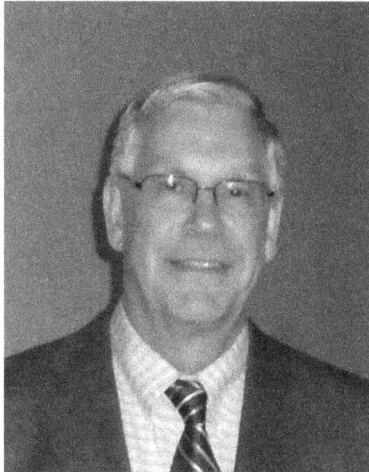

His work through the years earned him many awards. He was recognized as the Wisconsin Family Physician Educator of the Year in 1995. In 1996, he received the Patient Care Award for Innovation in Family Medicine Education presented at the National Society of Teachers of Family Medicine (STFM) in San Francisco, California for being co-concept originator and first editor of the Advanced Life Support in Obstetrics (ALSO) course. In 1997 he received the Distinguished Service Award from the Wisconsin State Medical Society, and he accepted the Rural Health Award from the Wisconsin Rural Health Cooperative in 2005. His patients nominated him for and he accepted the Wisconsin Family Physician of the Year award in 2006. Finally, he received the *Wisconsin Idea Award* presented on the University of Wisconsin–Madison campus in 2014 for his contributions to rural Wisconsin health. The Family Medicine Rural Training Program in Baraboo, Wisconsin to date has had an excellent track record placing doctors in rural communities who are also providing maternity care.

Dr. Damos is now retired from the practice of medicine and is caring for his wife, Linda, who is in the later stages of Alzheimer's disease. Anyone who knows him is aware that he has many more stories to tell beyond what has been shared in this book. He still enjoys storytelling to whoever will listen.

www.ingramcontent.com/pod-product-compliance
Lightning Source LLC
Chambersburg PA
CBHW031831090426
42741CB00005B/207